Diarmuid O'Donovan MD MSc FFPHMI DTM&H
is a medical doctor based in the west of Ireland.
He is Senior Lecturer in Social and Preventive Medicine
at the National University of Ireland, Galway
and a Director of Public Health in the Irish health service.
He has lived and worked in Sub-Saharan Africa and the UK,
and is involved in research and education on
health and development issues.

"Invaluable...I would not be without the complete set on my own shelves."
Times Educational Supplement

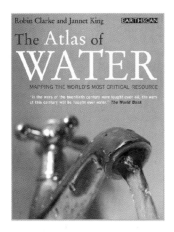

Robin Clarke and Jannet King — EARTHSCAN

The Atlas of WATER
MAPPING THE WORLD'S MOST CRITICAL RESOURCE

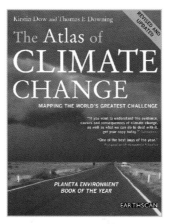

Kirstin Dow and Thomas E. Downing — REVISED AND UPDATED

The Atlas of CLIMATE CHANGE
MAPPING THE WORLD'S GREATEST CHALLENGE

PLANETA ENVIRONMENT BOOK OF THE YEAR

EARTHSCAN

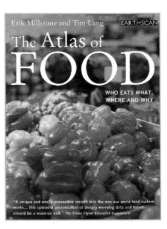

Erik Millstone and Tim Lang — EARTHSCAN

The Atlas of FOOD
WHO EATS WHAT, WHERE AND WHY

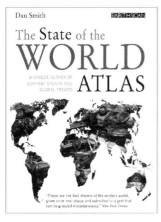

Dan Smith — EARTHSCAN

The State of the WORLD ATLAS
A UNIQUE SURVEY OF CURRENT EVENTS AND GLOBAL TRENDS

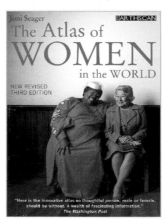

Joni Seager — EARTHSCAN

The Atlas of WOMEN in the WORLD
NEW REVISED THIRD EDITION

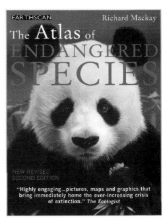

EARTHSCAN — Richard Mackay

The Atlas of ENDANGERED SPECIES
NEW REVISED SECOND EDITION
"Highly engaging...pictures, maps and graphics that bring immediately home the ever-increasing crisis of extinction." *The Ecologist*

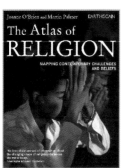

Joanne O'Brien and Martin Palmer — EARTHSCAN

The Atlas of RELIGION
MAPPING CONTEMPORARY CHALLENGES AND BELIEFS

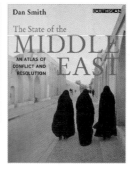

Dan Smith — EARTHSCAN

The State of the MIDDLE EAST
AN ATLAS OF CONFLICT AND RESOLUTION

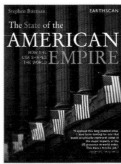

Stephen Burman — EARTHSCAN

The State of the AMERICAN EMPIRE
HOW THE USA SHAPES THE WORLD

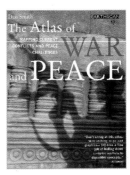

Dan Smith — EARTHSCAN

The Atlas of WAR and PEACE
MAPPING CURRENT CONFLICTS AND PEACE CHALLENGES

"No-one wishing to keep a grip on the reality of the world should be without these books." *International Herald Tribune*

"Fascinating and invaluable." *The Independent*

"A new kind of visual journalism." *New Scientist*

THE ATLAS OF

HEALTH

MAPPING THE CHALLENGES AND CAUSES OF DISEASE

DIARMUID O'DONOVAN

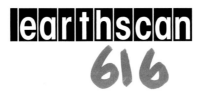

First published by Earthscan in the UK in 2008

A catalogue record for this book is available from the British Library

ISBN: 978-1-84407-465-5

Produced for Earthscan by
Myriad Editions
59 Lansdowne Place
Brighton, BN3 1FL, UK
www.MyriadEditions.com

Edited and coordinated by Jannet King and Candida Lacey
Designed by Isabelle Lewis and Corinne Pearlman
Maps and graphics created by Isabelle Lewis

Printed on paper produced from sustainable sources.
Printed and bound in Hong Kong through Lion Production
under the supervision of Bob Cassels, The Hanway Press, London

For a full list of publications please contact:

Earthscan
8–12 Camden High Street
London, NW1 0JH, UK
Tel: +44 (0)20 7387 8558
Fax: +44 (0)20 7387 8998
Email: earthinfo@earthscan.co.uk
Web: www.earthscan.co.uk

Earthscan publishes in association with
the International Institute for Environment and Development

CONTENTS

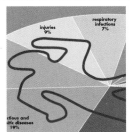

FOREWORD

"He who has not health has nothing."
French proverb

It was said recently that "if physicians were to read two articles per day of the 6 million medical articles published annually, in one year they would fall 82 centuries behind in their reading." These beautiful maps and graphics make the status of a wide range of health topics understandable at a glance, and will attract a much wider audience than would traditionally trawl through statistics in medical tomes and journals. This atlas will appeal alike to politicians, students, the media, health advocates – in fact, anyone concerned with the world's, or their nation's, health and medical services. Economics, poverty, inequality, education, climate, war – all impact on health, and the data presented here are vital to the planning of health services.

Since the first *State of Health Atlas* was published in 1993 there have been considerable improvements in health in some fields, but a disappointing and stubborn failure to improve in others. Infectious diseases, while diminishing, continue to challenge global health, with new and unexpected outbreaks around the corner. Chronic diseases such as cancer and heart disease are rising steadily, as a corollary to increasing longevity and risk factors such as obesity. As the world ages, the focus on prevention is timely.

A Chinese proverb states that "medicine can cure only curable diseases", and many of the health problems described here, especially the chronic diseases, will never be solved in the wards of hospitals, by curative care, or by expensive technology. They need to be addressed by individual action to improve health, encouraged and supported by political action such as government legislation on tobacco, alcohol, housing, or clean water supplies.

It is tempting to look back to when I proposed Myriad's first health atlas in the early 1990s. The World Health Organization considered there were insufficient data for such a publication, and the dearth of statistics was indeed a challenge. The atlas was written when computers were only just becoming widely used, and communication was much slower than it is today. The use of the internet to search by topic, by country, by year, by author, still lay some years ahead. We now not only have vastly improved health statistics, but also the means to research and collate them into a single book.

There is no publication other than this atlas that covers such diverse aspects of health, ranging from the personal to the political, from research to economics, from prevention to treatment, from youth to old age, and from a historical timeline to future challenges.

The atlas is a clarion call for targeted action – by governments, by individuals, by the whole of civil society.

Dr Judith Mackay
SBS, MBE, JP, MBChB (Edin), FRCP (Edin), FRCP (Lon)
Director of Global Tobacco Control Programmes, World Lung Foundation
TIME Magazine100: People Who Shape Our World 2007
Honorary Professor, Dept of Community Medicine, University of Hong Kong
Visiting Professor, Chinese Academy of Preventive Medicine

INTRODUCTION

"Do we not always find the diseases of the populace
traceable to defects in society?"
Rudolf Virchow (1821–1902)
Physician and public-health advocate

While great improvements in health have been seen in the last century, we are a long way from realizing the right of everyone to the "enjoyment of the highest attainable standard of physical and mental health" described in the International Bill of Human Rights.

A child born in Japan today can expect to live 82 years, while a child born in Swaziland can expect to live less than half as long: there, life expectancy is only 39 years. The probability of a child in Sierra Leone dying before the age of five is 282 in 1,000, whereas for a child born in Ireland the probability is five in 1,000. The differences are not only between countries. Within these countries, too, there are wide gaps between the health experience of the children of better-off parents and those of poor parents.

Health is defined by the World Health Organization as "a state of complete physical, mental and social well-being, not merely the absence of disease or infirmity". Other definitions include health as strength or ability and as the foundation for achievement of human potential. It is difficult to quantify health, well-being and disease, but where data do exist we have gathered the latest available to map the more measurable aspects of health and disease, and the factors that influence them, in order to provide a graphic picture of the state of global health.

Many economic, social, political and environmental factors influence levels of health, disease, disability and death. Experiences in early life, food and nutrition, work, unemployment, stress, social status, social support and social exclusion are key determinants. Major changes in the patterns of disease and causes of premature death in a population have less to do with advances in clinical medicine than with changes in environmental, social, political and economic conditions; improvements in women's social and education status; changes in agriculture and the availability of food; and preventive policy interventions in health and other sectors that have an impact on lifestyle, behaviour and work. The dramatic improvements in health in developed countries over the last 150 years are mainly due to improved living and working conditions, and the more democratic ways in which society has been organized; only recently have advances in medicine and healthcare played a major role. For example, deaths from tuberculosis in England and Wales declined even before the discovery of specific drugs for the disease.

Poverty is the central determinant of health, and reducing poverty will improve health outcomes. Poverty underlies most malnutrition, including obesity. It fuels the spread of many diseases, and increases the vulnerability to ill-health and trauma. Inadequate resources for public services lead to poor health and social services, which worsen the effects of poverty in households and communities. Addressing poverty is therefore essential to improving health. Every day, as health workers deal with the effects of hunger, food insecurity and unhealthy diets, lack of clean water and sanitation, inadequate education and illiteracy, environmental degradation and the underlying social and cultural contexts that influence these issues, they are involved in addressing poverty and its consequences.

Measuring health and poverty, and the effects of each, are fraught with difficulty, and never more so than in the poorest countries, poorest regions and among the poorest people; these are the places where relevant information is hardest to collect, analyze and use. A difference in the quality of data from different sources means there are limitations in comparability. Birth and death registration data from many countries are incomplete. High-quality data on the cause of death exist in systems that cover only 13 percent of the world's population. A further problem is that when data do exist, the way in which they are sorted, or aggregated, frequently hides sex and ethnic differences, as well as differences between regions, geographic areas, and urban and rural populations within a country. There are many limitations to statistics on health and its determinants. They are only as good as the ability of information systems to provide accurate and timely data. Because of these constraints, the information presented needs to be interpreted with caution.

In 2005, the World Health Organization established the Commission on the Social Determinants of Health to focus attention on evidence-based ways of creating better social conditions for health, especially for the world's most vulnerable people. The Commission is focusing on the causes of the causes, the social structures and the "socially determined conditions these create in which people grow, live, work and age". Recommendations for action will be made in the final report in 2008.

Health Inequity
Equity is an ethical concept of social justice, fairness and human rights, in which need rather than privilege is considered the appropriate foundation for the allocation of resources. Health inequalities are differences in health experiences and health outcomes between groups of people, according to socio-economic status, geographical area, age, sex, ethnicity and disability. Avoidable, unfair inequalities may be considered as inequities and, as such, as unacceptable.

Inequities describe differences in opportunity for different populations, which result in unequal life chances. The gradients in health and rates of mortality between the better-off and the poorest and most disadvantaged throughout the world are both avoidable and unacceptable. Development is described by Amartya Sen, the Nobel prize-winning economist, as the freedom to lead the life one has reason to value. He describes the lack of freedom associated with poverty, which robs people of the freedom to have clean water, adequate food and access to healthcare.

Income inequality within and between wealthy and poorer countries is growing. A high level of income inequality within a country has significant associations with lower life expectancy, higher rates of infant mortality and suicide, and with a decline in social cohesion and political engagement.

Gender inequality leads to health inequity, as is starkly demonstrated by the increasing rates of HIV infection in women in parts of Sub-Saharan Africa, where early and forced marriage, rape and sexual violence, lack of access to education, earning power and productive resources increase their vulnerability to infection. Understanding power and power relations in society is essential to addressing inequities in health and education to relieve poverty.

Health and Human Rights

Health and human rights are inextricably linked. The right to "the highest attainable standard of physical and mental health" and the right to "a standard of living adequate for the health and well-being of themselves and their family, including medical care, social services and security in the event of sickness, disability and old age", expressed in the International Bill of Human Rights, place a duty on governments to promote and protect the health of individuals and communities, including ensuring access to high-quality healthcare. Because economic, social, cultural and civil rights are interrelated, states are responsible for correcting conditions that prevent people realizing their right to health, as well as the related rights to education, safe living and working conditions, and freedom from discrimination. The right to the highest attainable standard of health includes globally legitimized standards, legal obligations on duty holders, and mechanisms of accountability, which require information systems, indicators and benchmarks to be able to describe and monitor the progressive realization of rights.

Governments provide the political, social and economic arrangements that determine whether rights are fulfilled. Governments that allow corruption or inappropriate public expenditure on armaments when large sections of the population are without access to the basic means of survival may be seen as committing human rights violations.

Globalization and Health

Globalization has both positive and negative implications for health and health inequities. Many improvements in disease treatment, prevention and surveillance have been organized on a global scale. But globalization can also pose risks to health through unfair trade and its regulation, the growing trend towards privatization of healthcare, the global pandemic of obesity, poorly managed migration, and the damage to the environment that is leading to climate change, with its potentially catastrophic associated effects on human health.

Trade agreements influenced by transnational corporations in the food, tobacco and pharmaceutical industries have a direct effect on public policy, which in turn affects the determinants of health. The Trade Related Aspects of Intellectual Property Rights (TRIPS) is designed to protect the rights of patent holders over new products, including drugs. In 2001 the World Trade Organization agreed that TRIPS should be implemented in a manner that supports the rights of countries "to protect public health and in particular to promote access to medicine for all", but there have been great difficulties in putting this into practice and, in particular, in developing and promoting the capacity of low- and middle-income countries to manufacture generic medicines.

While aid, or Official Development Assistance (ODA), is rising slowly, overall the amount of money returned to high-income countries in debt repayments from poorer countries far exceeds the amount given as aid. Servicing debt can cripple a nation's health, and damage developing health services. By 2007, only five high-income countries (Sweden, Luxembourg, Norway, Netherlands, Denmark) had reached the UN target of their overseas aid being at least 0.7 percent of gross national income.

Public Health and Reorienting Health Services

The term "public health" can refer to health systems, activities to improve health, or a movement. In 1988 the US Institute of Medicine defined the mission of public health as: "fulfilling society's interest in assuring conditions in which people can be healthy". In the UK, the most recent definition of public health is:

> The science and art of preventing disease, prolonging life and promoting health through the organized efforts and informed choices of society, organizations, public and private, communities and individuals.

Throughout the atlas, we have interpreted public health as actions to improve the health of populations and address health inequities.

In 2001, the Commission on Macroeconomics and Health estimated that $34 per person per year would supply essential interventions against infectious diseases and nutritional deficiencies, and increase the access of the world's poorest to essential services. Up to 2.1 billion people remain without access to essential medicines, 80 percent of whom live in low-income countries. Essential medicines are those that satisfy the priority healthcare needs of the population. They are intended to be available at all times in the context of functioning health systems – in adequate amounts, in the appropriate dosage forms, with assured quality and adequate information, at an affordable price. Annual expenditure per person on medicines in 2000 varied from $396 in the USA to $4 in low-income countries, even though medicines accounted for a higher percentage of health expenditure in low- and middle-income countries than in high-income countries.

Comprehensive primary healthcare (PHC) is central to improving health. Often misrepresented as the primary level of the health service, the principles of PHC aim to promote and protect good health as well as cure disease; integrate different services to work together; address neglected and marginalized populations; use health technologies appropriately and in ways that are socially and culturally acceptable; be community-driven and human-rights focused.

Improving Global Health

The eight Millennium Development Goals agreed by the United Nations General Assembly in September 2000 all include elements that address health either directly or indirectly. Achieving the first development goal – to eradicate extreme poverty and hunger – would have more impact on improving global health status than any other measure.

Poverty remains the most important cause of ill-health because it involves poor nutrition, lack of safe water, poor education, poor housing and poor access to effective health services. The vast majority of premature deaths and preventable illness and disability occur in the less-developed, less-resourced, poorer nations and regions of the world. Despite the knowledge of cost-effective interventions, few of these have been implemented and the burden of disease falls unduly on poor people and societies.

This book grew out of lectures given to students from a range of disciplines on health as experienced by people around the world, and from using other atlases in the series to demonstrate global differences in health and its determinants. The topics covered here have been chosen to give an introduction to the avoidable gross inequities in health that continue to grow between and within countries, and the ways in which health in every part of the world is affected by global changes. While it is not possible to address all of these topics in great detail, and some important subjects have not been covered, I hope that readers will be encouraged to explore further. People everywhere are more interconnected than ever before. As life expectancy and quality of life improve for the rich, millions are still dying for want of food, clean water, and affordable medicines. These gross inequities are unsustainable, and we all have a role to play in addressing them.

Diarmuid O'Donovan
November 2007

Acknowledgements
This atlas brings together information that people all over the world have collected, and which others have compiled into statistics. It comes from a range of sources, in particular the WHO, UNDP and UNICEF. Full details are given on pages 118–125.

My sincere thanks go to the team at Myriad Editions: Candida Lacey for instigating and leading this collaboration, and for guiding and advising at all stages; Jannet King for additional research and for scrupulous editing, checking, double-checking, advising, and patiently waiting for overdue work; Isabelle Lewis for finding dramatic ways of graphically illustrating the issues; and Corinne Pearlman for her creative direction and design input.

I would like to acknowledge Judith Mackay, who wrote the first *State of Health Atlas* and subsequent atlases of Tobacco, Cancer, and Heart Disease and Stroke that I use for teaching, and which inspired this whole endeavour.

Thanks go especially to my family – to Mary and to Annie, Katie and Oisín, who have patiently supported the development of this atlas.

LIFE EXPECTANCY AND POPULATION
1950 and 2005

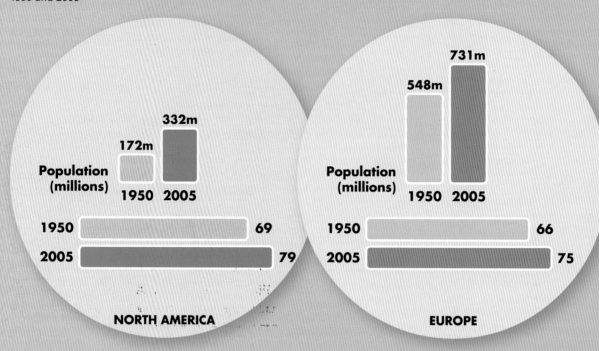

NORTH AMERICA

Population
(millions)

172m
1950

332m
2005

1950 69
2005 79

EUROPE

Population
(millions)

548m
1950

731m
2005

1950 66
2005 75

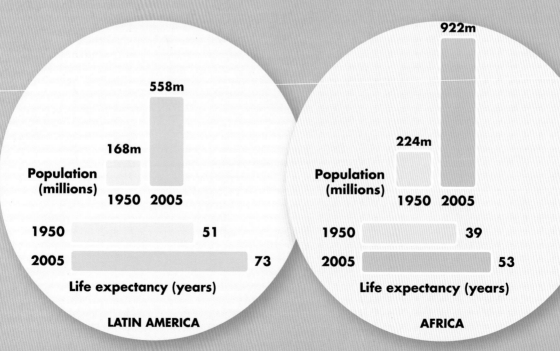

LATIN AMERICA

Population
(millions)

168m
1950

558m
2005

1950 51
2005 73

Life expectancy (years)

AFRICA

Population
(millions)

224m
1950

922m
2005

1950 39
2005 53

Life expectancy (years)

PART 1

A PICTURE OF HEALTH

There are clear links between the health of a population and a country's overall level of development. Since the 1950s, life expectancy has increased around the world, in some countries very dramatically, as a result of improvements in living and working conditions, the ways in which society has been organized, and advances in medicine and healthcare.

Life expectancy is lowest where child and maternal mortality rates are still high, and communicable diseases are the most common cause of premature death. Fertility rates are also very high in these regions, as is clear from the massive increase in population that has taken place over the last half century. A key element to reducing both premature mortality and family size is to educate girls, enabling them to grow into women equipped with the skills, income, and knowledge about contraception to make choices that will lead to smaller, healthier families.

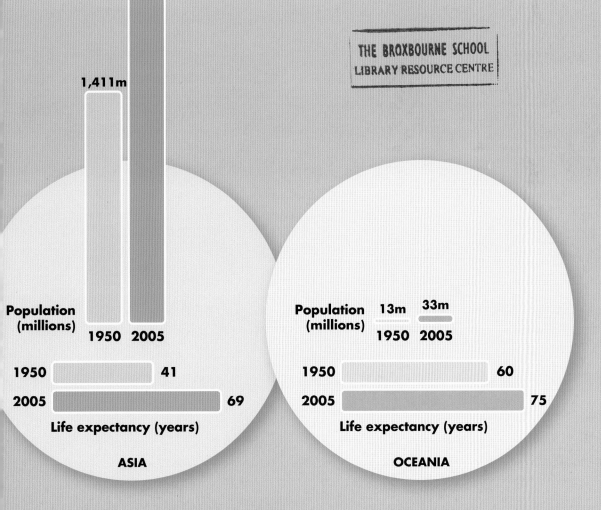

ASIA

3,938m

1,411m

Population (millions)

1950   2005

| 1950 | | 41 |
| 2005 | | 69 |

Life expectancy (years)

OCEANIA

Population (millions)

13m   33m

1950   2005

| 1950 | | 60 |
| 2005 | | 75 |

Life expectancy (years)

Life expectancy is increasing in most countries, but is declining in southern Africa.

Life expectancy at birth is an assessment of the average number of years newborn infants can expect to live, based on current conditions. Worldwide, people can expect to live longer than at any time in history. Clean water, better nutrition, improved housing and working conditions, and access to appropriate health services are the main influences. In every country, wealthier people live longer than poor people, and in most populations women can expect to live longer than men.

Low life expectancy tends to reflect child death rates, and the level of control of the communicable diseases that affect young children (such as respiratory infections and diarrhoeal disease). The populations of countries with a low life expectancy and a high proportion of young people (under 15) are especially vulnerable. If people survive the early years, their life expectancy usually improves.

The recent decline in life expectancy in many countries in Sub-Saharan Africa is related to the HIV/AIDS epidemic. In some countries of the former Soviet Union life expectancy has also declined during the transition from communism, and the subsequent changes in social and economic conditions. Health appears to have improved in the former communist states that have embraced democracy most enthusiastically.

LIFE EXPECTANCY
Predicted life-span
for a child born in 2003
2005

■ under 40 years		60 – 69 years	
■ 40 – 49 years		70 years and over	
50 – 59 years		no data	

⬤ 40% or more people are aged under 15 years
2005

CANADA

USA

MEXICO

BAHAMAS
CUBA
DOMINICAN REP.
JAMAICA   HAITI   PUERTO RICO
BELIZE   VIRGIN IS. (US)
GUATEMALA   HONDURAS
EL SALVADOR   NICARAGUA
COSTA RICA
PANAMA

GUADELOUPE
ST LUCIA   MARTINIQUE
N. ANTILLES   BARBADOS
ST VINCENT & GRENADINES
TRINIDAD & TOBAGO
VENEZUELA   GUYANA
SURINAME
COLOMBIA   FRENCH GUIANA

ECUADOR

PERU

BRAZIL

BOLIVIA

CHILE   PARAGUAY

URUGUAY

ARGENTINA

WE
SA
CAPE VERDE   M
SENEGAL
GAMBIA
GUINEA-   GU
BISSAU   SIERR
LIBER

Chile, Mexico, Tunisia and India have seen greatest improvement in life expectancy since 1950.

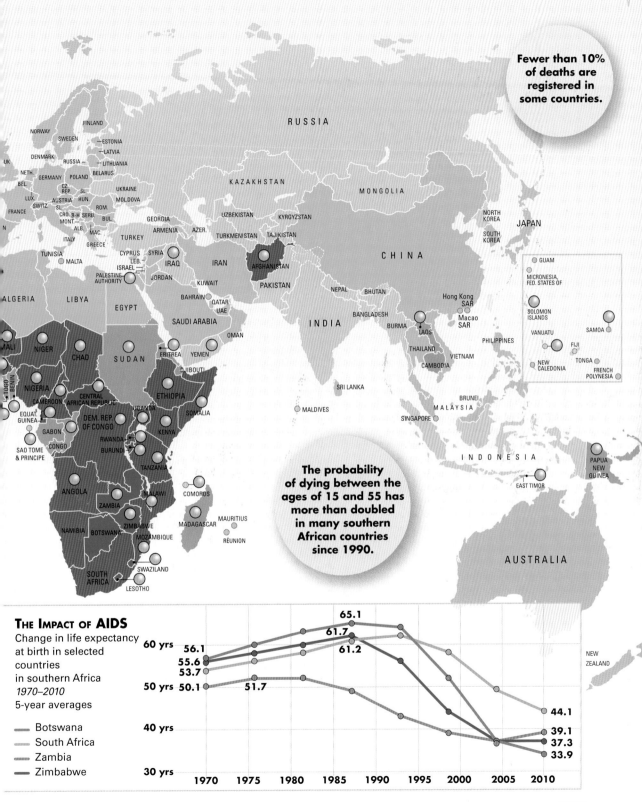

Fewer than 10% of deaths are registered in some countries.

The probability of dying between the ages of 15 and 55 has more than doubled in many southern African countries since 1990.

THE IMPACT OF AIDS

Change in life expectancy at birth in selected countries in southern Africa
1970–2010
5-year averages

— Botswana
— South Africa
— Zambia
— Zimbabwe

65.1
61.7
61.2
56.1
55.6
53.7
50.1
51.7
44.1
39.1
37.3
33.9

60 yrs
50 yrs
40 yrs
30 yrs

1970 1975 1980 1985 1990 1995 2000 2005 2010

Every minute a woman dies from complications related to pregnancy or childbirth.

The direct causes of maternal deaths are the same all over the world: severe bleeding, infections, hypertension (causing eclampsia and convulsions), prolonged or obstructed labour, and complications arising from unsafe abortions.

Death in pregnancy and childbirth are rare in wealthy countries. Factors that influence the risk of women dying during or shortly after pregnancy include poor health before pregnancy, inadequate, inappropriate, inaccessible or unaffordable healthcare, and poor hygiene and care during childbirth. Related to all of these are poverty, low levels of education and illiteracy, and gender-based social rules, including women's unequal access to resources and their lack of decision-making power in families and societies.

Programmes that promote "safe motherhood" aim to create circumstances whereby a pregnant woman receives care for the prevention, detection and treatment of pregnancy complications, a woman in labour has access to skilled birth assistance, and, if a mother and her newborn need it, they have access to emergency obstetric care, and care after birth.

MATERNAL MORTALITY
Number of women who die in pregnancy or childbirth per 100,000 live births
2000

■	1,000 or more		10 – 99
▨	500 – 999		fewer than 10
▨	100 – 499	▨	no data

Percentage of births not attended by a doctor, nurse or midwife

Ⓧ 75% or more

◯ 50% – 74%

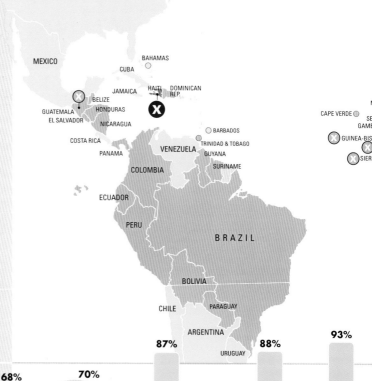

ANTENATAL CARE
Percentage of women attended at least once during pregnancy by skilled health personnel
1997–2005

- **53%** South Asia
- **68%** Sub-Saharan Africa
- **70%** Middle East & North Africa
- **87%** Eastern Europe, Russia & Central Asia
- **88%** East Asia & Pacific
- **93%** Latin America & Caribbean

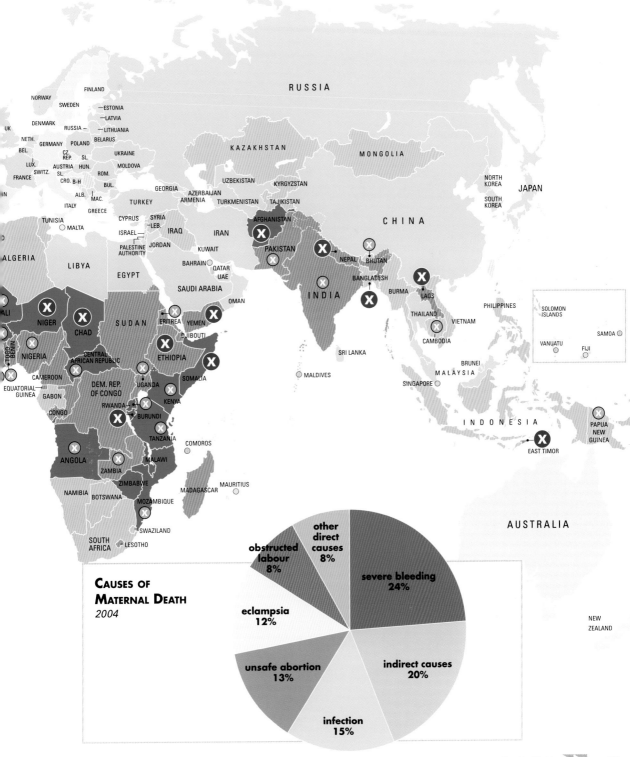

CAUSES OF
MATERNAL DEATH
2004

- other direct causes 8%
- obstructed labour 8%
- eclampsia 12%
- unsafe abortion 13%
- severe bleeding 24%
- indirect causes 20%
- infection 15%

Child deaths account for about one-fifth of all deaths occurring annually in the world.

Child death rates are declining globally, but have increased in some countries. They are closely linked to poverty, with most occurring in poor countries. A child in a developing country is 12 times more likely to die before the age of five than a child in a developed country.

Almost four in 10 child deaths occur in the first four weeks of life, the neonatal period. Most of these deaths could be prevented with affordable low-technology solutions, such as tetanus toxoid immunization for the mother during pregnancy, clean delivery kits, including a sterile blade to cut the umbilical cord, immediate and exclusive breastfeeding, drying and warming the baby immediately after birth, and early postnatal checkups.

Five infectious diseases (pneumonia, diarrhoea, malaria, measles and HIV/AIDS) cause half of the deaths of under-fives, and malnutrition is an underlying factor.

Low-cost treatments and high-impact preventive interventions such as micronutrient supplements, antibiotics, immunization and bednets to prevent mosquito bites are helping to reduce child deaths.

In rich countries, new problems are emerging in child health. Diet and physical inactivity contribute to the growing epidemic of child obesity, which leads to major health problems, both in childhood and later life.

In all countries children from wealthier households are less likely to die: they have better levels of nutrition and education, fewer injuries and higher levels of healthcare use, including immunization.

CHILD DEATH RATE

Under-five mortality rate
per 1,000 live births
2005

- 250 or more
- 175 – 249
- 100 – 174
- 25 – 99
- 10 – 24
- fewer than 10
- no data

↑ under-five mortality rate increased or remained the same *1990–2005*

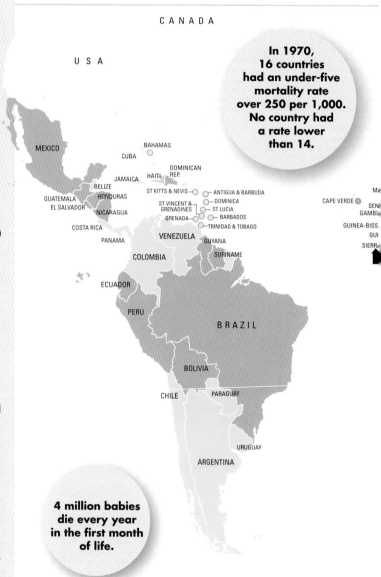

In 1970, 16 countries had an under-five mortality rate over 250 per 1,000. No country had a rate lower than 14.

4 million babies die every year in the first month of life.

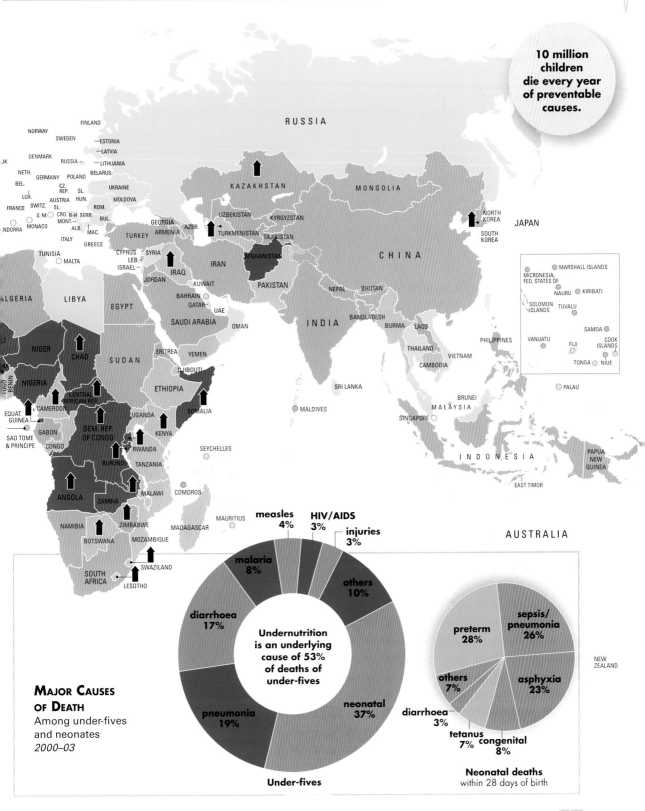

10 million children die every year of preventable causes.

RUSSIA

NORWAY
SWEDEN
FINLAND
—ESTONIA
—LATVIA
RUSSIA —
—LITHUANIA
BELARUS
DENMARK
NETH.
GERMANY POLAND
BEL.
LUX.
CZ. REP. SL.
AUSTRIA HUN.
SWITZ. SL.
FRANCE
S.M.
MONT.—
ANDORRA MONACO
ITALY
ALB.
MAC.
GREECE

UKRAINE
MOLDOVA
ROM.
CRO. B-H SERB.
BUL.

KAZAKHSTAN
MONGOLIA

GEORGIA
ARMENIA AZER.
TURKEY
UZBEKISTAN
KYRGYZSTAN
TURKMENISTAN
TAJIKISTAN

CYPRUS
LEB.—
SYRIA
ISRAEL —
IRAQ
JORDAN
KUWAIT
BAHRAIN
QATAR
UAE

IRAN
AFGHANISTAN

CHINA

PAKISTAN
NEPAL
BHUTAN

NORTH KOREA
JAPAN
SOUTH KOREA

TUNISIA
MALTA

ALGERIA
LIBYA
EGYPT
SAUDI ARABIA
OMAN

INDIA
BANGLADESH
BURMA
LAOS

NIGER
CHAD
SUDAN
ERITREA
YEMEN
DJIBOUTI
ETHIOPIA
SOMALIA

THAILAND
VIETNAM
CAMBODIA

NIGERIA
BENIN
CAMEROON
CENTRAL AFRICAN REP.
UGANDA
KENYA
EQUAT. GUINEA
GABON
SAO TOME & PRINCIPE
CONGO
DEM. REP. OF CONGO
RWANDA
BURUNDI
TANZANIA

SRI LANKA
MALDIVES

ANGOLA
ZAMBIA
MALAWI
COMOROS
MAURITIUS

SEYCHELLES

BRUNEI
MALAYSIA
SINGAPORE

INDONESIA

PAPUA NEW GUINEA

EAST TIMOR

NAMIBIA
ZIMBABWE
BOTSWANA
MOZAMBIQUE
MADAGASCAR

SOUTH AFRICA
SWAZILAND
LESOTHO

MARSHALL ISLANDS
MICRONESIA, FED. STATES OF
NAURU KIRIBATI
SOLOMON ISLANDS
TUVALU
SAMOA
VANUATU
FIJI
COOK ISLANDS
TONGA NIUE
PALAU

PHILIPPINES

AUSTRALIA

NEW ZEALAND

MAJOR CAUSES OF DEATH
Among under-fives and neonates
2000–03

Under-fives

Undernutrition is an underlying cause of 53% of deaths of under-fives

- measles 4%
- HIV/AIDS 3%
- injuries 3%
- others 10%
- malaria 8%
- diarrhoea 17%
- pneumonia 19%
- neonatal 37%

Neonatal deaths
within 28 days of birth

- preterm 28%
- sepsis/pneumonia 26%
- asphyxia 23%
- others 7%
- diarrhoea 3%
- tetanus 7%
- congenital 8%

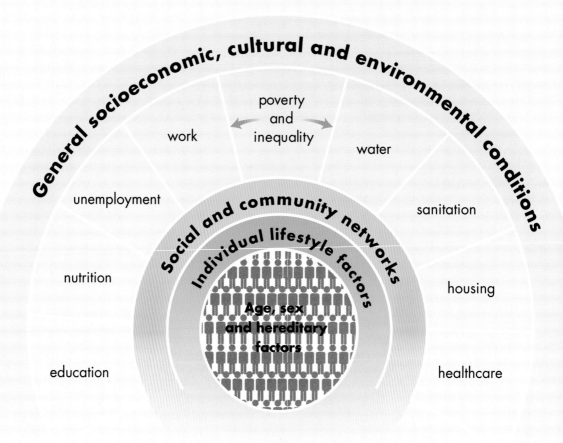

General socioeconomic, cultural and environmental conditions

poverty
and
inequality

work

water

unemployment

Social and community networks

Individual lifestyle factors

sanitation

nutrition

Age, sex
and hereditary
factors

housing

education

healthcare

PART 2

DETERMINANTS OF HEALTH

The factors that can have positive or negative effects on health have been described as "layers of influence". There is very little we can do about our age, sex or genetic makeup, but aspects of our lifestyle – including whether or not we smoke, our level of physical activity and our choice of diet – and the influence of our peers and the community in which we live all impact on our health.

Our ability to maintain good health and wellbeing is determined to a great extent by the conditions in which we live and work, which are, in turn, strongly influenced by the level of poverty and inequality in society. These wider economic, cultural and environmental conditions affect health at a population level.

Many of the social and economic factors that influence our health can be changed by global, national and local policies – that is, by the policies that influence political, commercial and individual decisions.

Wealth influences health.

The health of the populations of poor countries is worse than that of rich countries, and the health of wealthier people everywhere is better than that of poor people.

Material deprivation affects all the determinants of health, including food, water and sanitation, education, and access to public services. The Human Poverty Index scores developing countries according to life expectancy, adult literacy, access to safe water, and underweight children, and can be an indicator of poor health outcomes.

Gross National Income (GNI), which may be used to demonstrate the average wealth of an economy, correlates with life expectancy, maternal and child mortality, and education enrolment, but it does not show internal differences, such as disparities between socio-economic or racial/ethnic groups, or between regions within a country. Inequality ratios compare the income of the richest and the poorest citizens of a country. There is a strong correlation between unequal societies and poor health outcomes.

Many countries do not have information systems that allow data to be analyzed by social position, but in countries where this has been investigated, wide differences are seen in the health of different socio-economic groups in both rich and poor countries. The countries with the highest life expectancy and lowest infant mortality tend to be those where income is more evenly distributed, as in Canada, Japan and Norway.

Poverty is more than a lack of money. It means not participating fully in society, and having limits on leading the life one has reason to value. Addressing poverty includes addressing opportunity, empowerment, security and dignity.

HEALTH AND POVERTY

Infant deaths
per 1,000 live births
2005

- 150 or more
- 100 – 149
- 50 – 99
- 10 – 49
- fewer than 10
- no data

15 countries with worst Human Poverty Index score

GNI per capita less than $350

income of richest 20% more than 25 times that of poorest 20%

CANADA

USA

MEXICO

BAHAMAS
CUBA
JAMAICA HAITI DOMINICAN REP.
BELIZE
GUATEMALA HONDURAS
EL SALVADOR
NICARAGUA
COSTA RICA
PANAMA

ST KITTS & NEVIS
ST VINCENT & GRENADINES
GRENADA

ANTIGUA & BARBUDA
DOMINICA
ST LUCIA
BARBADOS
TRINIDAD & TOBAGO

VENEZUELA GUYANA
SURINAME
COLOMBIA

ECUADOR

PERU

BRAZIL

BOLIVIA

CHILE PARAGUAY

ARGENTINA

URUGUAY

CAPE VERDE M
SE
GAMBIA
GUINEA-BISS
GUI
SIERRA

CHILD MORTALITY AND POVERTY

Under-five mortality rates
per 1,000 children
latest data available 1990–2001
selected countries
within World Bank regions

- 20% of population with lowest income
- 20% of population with highest income

Life Expectancy 16–17; Maternal Health 18–19; Child Health 20–21

POVERTY AND INEQUALITY

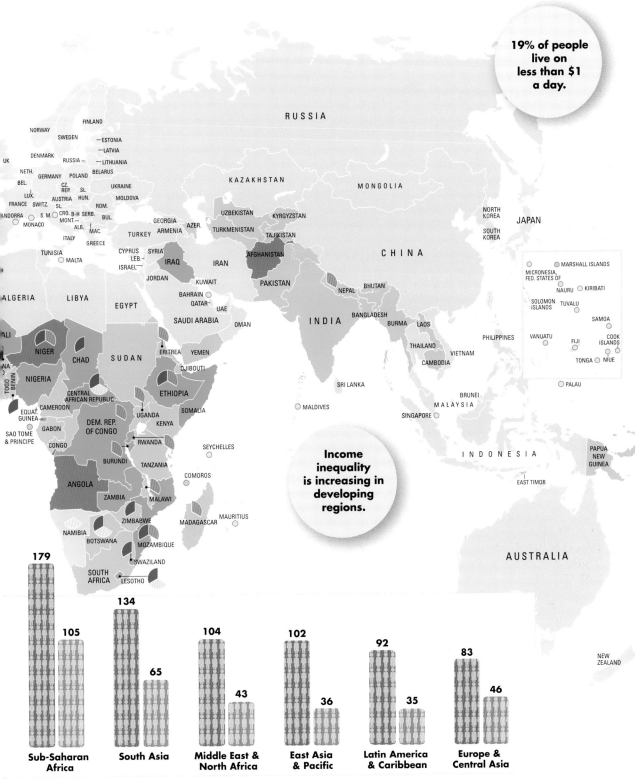

19% of people live on less than $1 a day.

Income inequality is increasing in developing regions.

RUSSIA

NORWAY
FINLAND
SWEDEN
ESTONIA
LATVIA
DENMARK
RUSSIA —
LITHUANIA
UK
BELARUS
NETH.
GERMANY POLAND
BEL.
CZ.
REP. SL.
UKRAINE
LUX.
AUSTRIA HUN.
MOLDOVA
FRANCE SWITZ. SL.
ROM.
ANDORRA
S. M. CRO. B-H SERB.
BUL.
MONACO
MONT. ALB.
MAC.
ITALY
GREECE

KAZAKHSTAN
MONGOLIA

NORTH
KOREA
JAPAN
SOUTH
KOREA

TUNISIA
MALTA
CYPRUS
LEB.
ISRAEL
SYRIA
IRAQ
IRAN
JORDAN
TURKEY
GEORGIA
ARMENIA AZER.
TURKMENISTAN
UZBEKISTAN
KYRGYZSTAN
TAJIKISTAN
AFGHANISTAN

CHINA

ALGERIA
LIBYA
EGYPT
KUWAIT
BAHRAIN
QATAR
UAE
SAUDI ARABIA
OMAN
PAKISTAN
NEPAL BHUTAN
INDIA
BANGLADESH
BURMA
LAOS

MARSHALL ISLANDS
MICRONESIA,
FED. STATES OF
NAURU KIRIBATI
SOLOMON
ISLANDS
TUVALU
SAMOA
VANUATU
FIJI
COOK
ISLANDS
TONGA NIUE
PALAU

MALI
NIGER
CHAD
SUDAN
ERITREA
YEMEN
DJIBOUTI
NIGERIA
CENTRAL
AFRICAN REPUBLIC
ETHIOPIA
SOMALIA
TOGO
BENIN
EQUAT.
GUINEA
CAMEROON
UGANDA
KENYA
SAO TOME
& PRINCIPE
GABON
DEM. REP.
OF CONGO
CONGO
RWANDA
BURUNDI
TANZANIA

THAILAND
VIETNAM
CAMBODIA
PHILIPPINES

SRI LANKA
MALDIVES

BRUNEI
MALAYSIA
SINGAPORE

PAPUA
NEW
GUINEA

SEYCHELLES
COMOROS

INDONESIA

EAST TIMOR

ANGOLA
ZAMBIA
MALAWI
NAMIBIA
ZIMBABWE
MADAGASCAR
MAURITIUS
BOTSWANA
MOZAMBIQUE
SWAZILAND
SOUTH
AFRICA
LESOTHO

AUSTRALIA

NEW
ZEALAND

179 Sub-Saharan Africa — 105

134 South Asia — 65

104 Middle East & North Africa — 43

102 East Asia & Pacific — 36

92 Latin America & Caribbean — 35

83 Europe & Central Asia — 46

Education, particularly of girls and women, has a direct bearing on health.

Women's education is the strongest instrument available for reducing infant mortality and child malnutrition. Literate women are more likely to immunize their children, and female education reduces the risk of maternal death, increases birth spacing and improves nutrition of women and children.

Education is called the "social vaccine" against HIV/AIDS. Children who complete their primary education are likely to know more about the disease, including information on how to protect themselves against it.

The burden of illiteracy, like that of ill-health, falls mainly on poor women. There is a huge disparity in access to education between the richest and poorest within countries, and inequality in the educational attainment of girls and boys has been shown to adversely affect child mortality.

Lack of education can lead to ill-health and, conversely, poor health has a negative impact on education. Respiratory infections, diarrhoea, malaria, TB and HIV/AIDS keep millions of children and teachers away from school. In order for educational opportunities to be increased in the poorest countries, millions more trained teachers are needed, especially female teachers.

FEMALE EDUCATION AND CHILD SURVIVAL
Percentage of girls of the appropriate age enrolled in primary school *2004*

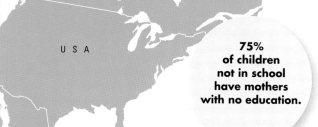

- under 50%
- 50% – 69%
- 70% – 89%
- 90% or more
- no data

- under-five mortality rate is 150 or more per 1,000 live births *2005*
- girls' participation in primary education is less than 80% that of boys' *2004*

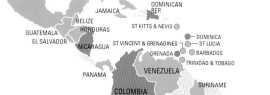

CANADA

USA

75% of children not in school have mothers with no education.

MEXICO

BAHAMAS
CUBA
JAMAICA
DOMINICAN REP.
BELIZE
HONDURAS
ST KITTS & NEVIS
GUATEMALA
EL SALVADOR
NICARAGUA
ST VINCENT & GRENADINES
DOMINICA
ST LUCIA
GRENADA
BARBADOS
TRINIDAD & TOBAGO
PANAMA
VENEZUELA
SURINAME
COLOMBIA

M
CAPE VERDE
SEN
GAMBI
GUINEA-BISSAU
GUINEA
SIERRA LEONE
LIBERIA

ECUADOR

PERU

Two-thirds of illiterate adults are women.

BOLIVIA

ARGENTINA

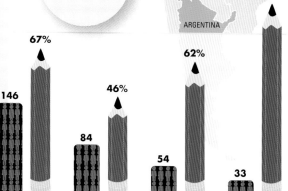

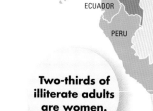

LITERACY SAVES LIVES
2005

- number of deaths of under-fives per 1,000 live births
- percentage of women who are literate

190 / 38%	146 / 67%	84 / 46%	54 / 62%	33 / 87%	31 / 90%
West & Central Africa	**Eastern & Southern Africa**	**South Asia**	**Middle East & North Africa**	**East Asia & Pacific**	**Latin America & Caribbean**

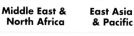 *Maternal Health 18–19; Child Health 20–21*

EDUCATION

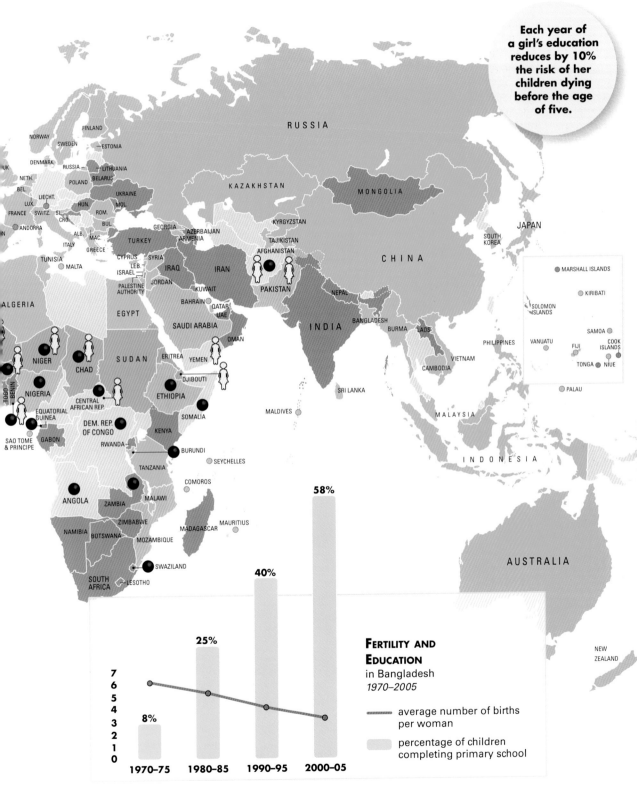

Each year of a girl's education reduces by 10% the risk of her children dying before the age of five.

FERTILITY AND EDUCATION
in Bangladesh
1970–2005

— — — average number of births per woman

percentage of children completing primary school

8% — 1970–75
25% — 1980–85
40% — 1990–95
58% — 2000–05

Malnutrition is the most important worldwide cause of ill-health and death.

Undernutrition weakens a person's ability to fight infection, and therefore increases the incidence, severity and duration of diseases. It accounts for 12 percent of deaths worldwide, and in developing countries 60 percent of deaths in under-fives are associated with the children having a low weight for their age. Malnourished people are also at increased risk of diarrhoeal disease from contaminated food and water; diarrhoea worsens the effects of malnutrition.

Overnutrition, specifically diets that include large amounts of energy-dense, nutrient-poor foods that are high in fat, sugar and salt, contributes to the development of heart disease, stroke, diabetes and certain cancers. These risks are increased by low levels of physical activity and tobacco use. Low intake of fruit and vegetables is estimated to contribute to 31 percent of heart disease, 11 percent of stroke and 19 percent of gastrointestinal cancer. Changes in oral disease patterns are closely related to changes in diet, tobacco use and alcohol.

Undernutrition is not caused by a global shortage of food. There is more than enough food to go round. It is associated with poverty. Poor children are the most likely to be underweight at birth. Better maternal nutrition improves the likelihood of both mother and child surviving. Improved child survival reduces population growth.

Good nutrition is a foundation for many development goals, especially for those relating to health, education, gender equality and poverty alleviation.

DENTAL CARIES
Average number of decayed, missing or filled teeth in 12-year-olds
2004
WHO regions

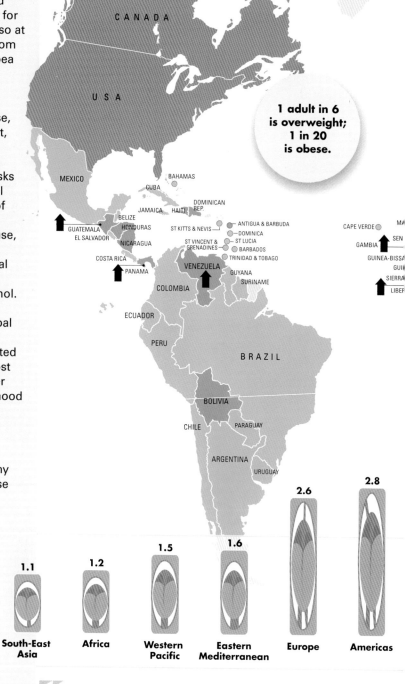

CALORIFIC INTAKE
Average kCal per person per day
2001–03

- less than 2,000
- 2,001 – 2,500
- 2,501 – 3,000
- 3,001 – 3,500
- more than 3,500
- no data

↑ increase of 50% or more in number of undernourished people between 1990–92 (1993–95 for Europe and Central Asia) and 2001–03

1 adult in 6 is overweight; 1 in 20 is obese.

South-East Asia 1.1
Africa 1.2
Western Pacific 1.5
Eastern Mediterranean 1.6
Europe 2.6
Americas 2.8

FOOD AND NUTRITION

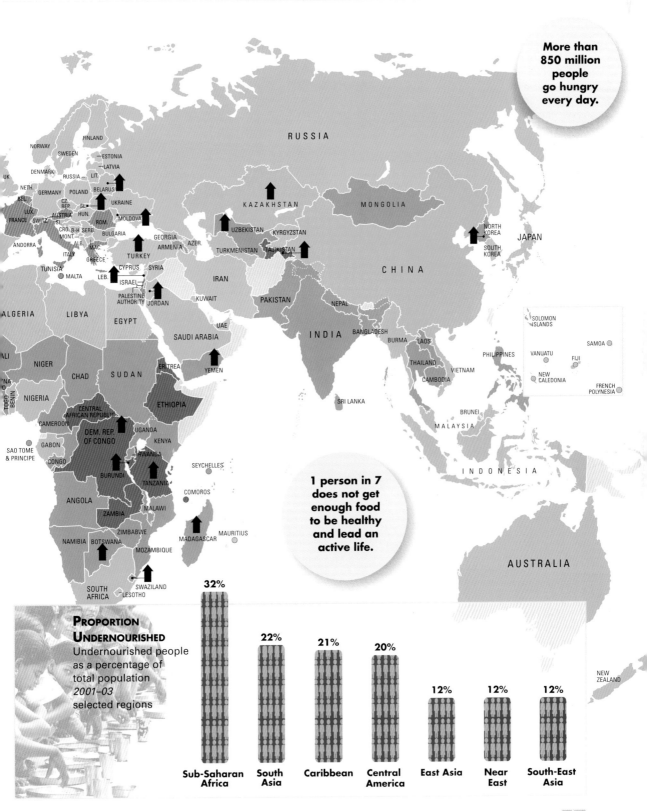

More than 850 million people go hungry every day.

RUSSIA

NORWAY
SWEDEN
FINLAND
DENMARK
UK
NETH.
BEL.
GERMANY
POLAND
LUX.
FRANCE
SWITZ.
ANDORRA
ITALY
TUNISIA
MALTA
RUSSIA
LIT.
ESTONIA
LATVIA
BELARUS
UKRAINE
MOLDOVA
CZ. REP.
SL.
AUSTRIA
HUN.
SL.
CRO.
B-H
MONT.
SERB.
ROM.
BULGARIA
MAC.
ALB.
GREECE
TURKEY
CYPRUS
LEB.
SYRIA
ISRAEL
PALESTINE AUTHORITY
JORDAN
GEORGIA
ARMENIA
AZER.

KAZAKHSTAN
UZBEKISTAN
KYRGYZSTAN
TURKMENISTAN
TAJIKISTAN

MONGOLIA

NORTH KOREA
SOUTH KOREA
JAPAN

CHINA

ALGERIA
LIBYA
EGYPT
MALI
NIGER
CHAD
SUDAN
NIGERIA
TOGO
BENIN
CAMEROON
CENTRAL AFRICAN REPUBLIC
DEM. REP. OF CONGO
GABON
CONGO
SAO TOME & PRINCIPE
UGANDA
KENYA
RWANDA
BURUNDI
TANZANIA
ANGOLA
ZAMBIA
MALAWI
NAMIBIA
BOTSWANA
ZIMBABWE
MOZAMBIQUE
SWAZILAND
LESOTHO
SOUTH AFRICA
SEYCHELLES
COMOROS
MADAGASCAR
MAURITIUS
ERITREA
ETHIOPIA
YEMEN
SAUDI ARABIA
UAE
KUWAIT
IRAN
IRAQ
PAKISTAN
NEPAL
INDIA
BANGLADESH
BURMA
SRI LANKA
LAOS
THAILAND
VIETNAM
CAMBODIA
PHILIPPINES
BRUNEI
MALAYSIA
INDONESIA

SOLOMON ISLANDS
VANUATU
SAMOA
FIJI
NEW CALEDONIA
FRENCH POLYNESIA

1 person in 7 does not get enough food to be healthy and lead an active life.

AUSTRALIA

NEW ZEALAND

PROPORTION UNDERNOURISHED
Undernourished people as a percentage of total population *2001–03* selected regions

32%
Sub-Saharan Africa

22%
South Asia

21%
Caribbean

20%
Central America

12%
East Asia

12%
Near East

12%
South-East Asia

Water and Sanitation 30–31; Heart Disease and Stroke 46–47; Diabetes 49–49; Urbanization 72–73; Unhealthy Diets 86–87

More than 1.1 billion people lack access to safe water, and 2.6 billion lack access to adequate sanitation.

Lack of safe water, sanitation and hygiene are major risk factors for disease and death, especially in children. Nearly 2 million people die each year as a result of diarrhoea and other diseases caused by ingesting contaminated water and not having access to adequate sanitation. Diarrhoea can lead to malnutrition, which increases the risk of death from disease.

Other waterborne infections, such as schistosomiasis, are transmitted through contact with infected water. Water contaminated by toxic chemicals such as arsenic also causes disease and death.

Supplies of adequate quantities of water are essential for personal and household hygiene, and a shortage can lead to the transmission of fly-borne diseases such as trachoma, the main preventable cause of blindness in developing countries.

Searching for and collecting water in rural areas is work done mainly by poor women and girls. The time spent doing this prevents them participating in education and income-generating employment. Poor families without access to safe water can become poorer through ill-health caused by contaminated water. Where people have to pay for water, the poorest often have to pay relatively more than wealthier people.

ACCESS TO WATER

Percentage of population with sustainable access to an improved water source
2004

- fewer than 50%
- 50% – 69%
- 70% – 89%
- 90% or more
- no data

◎ diarrhoeal diseases caused more than 100 deaths per 100,000 people *2002*

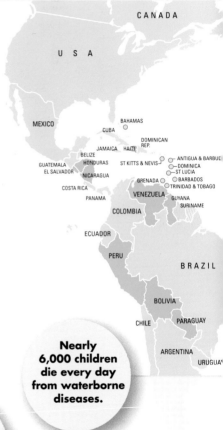

Nearly 6,000 children die every day from waterborne diseases.

88% of diarrhoeal disease is attributed to unsafe water supplies, inadequate sanitation and poor hygiene.

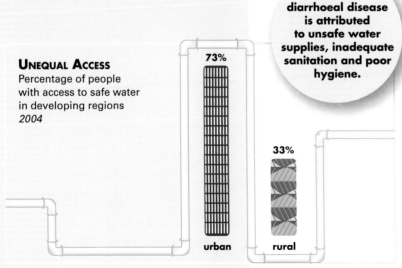

UNEQUAL ACCESS

Percentage of people with access to safe water in developing regions
2004

73% urban

33% rural

ACCESS TO SANITATION

Percentage of population with sustainable access to improved sanitation
2004

- fewer than 30%
- 30% – 49%
- 50% – 69%
- 70% – 89%
- 90% or more

Child Health 20–21; Food and Nutrition 28–29

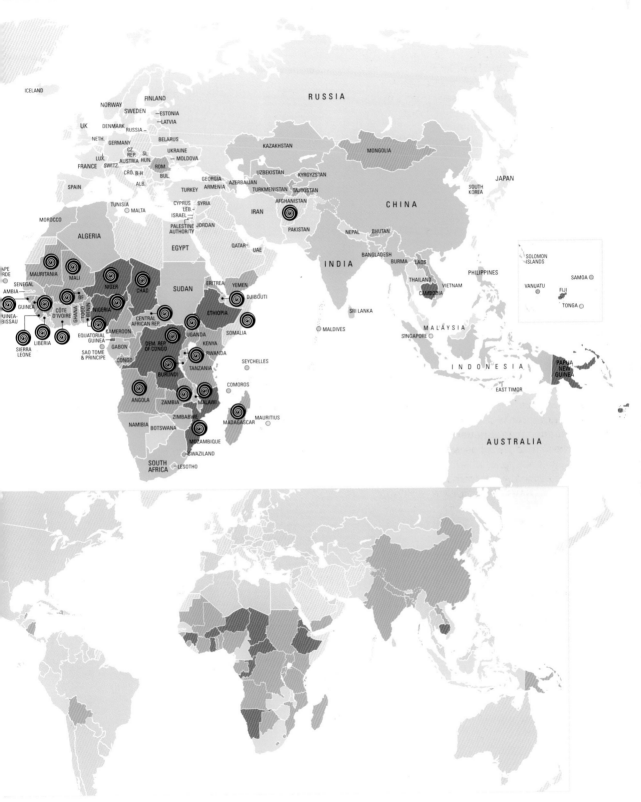

ICELAND

NORWAY   FINLAND   RUSSIA
     SWEDEN   ─ESTONIA
UK DENMARK RUSSIA ─   ─LATVIA
 NETH. GERMANY   BELARUS
   LUX. CZ SL   KAZAKHSTAN   MONGOLIA
FRANCE AUSTRIA HUN. UKRAINE
   SWITZ.   ROM. ─MOLDOVA   JAPAN
SPAIN   CRO. B-H BUL.   UZBEKISTAN KYRGYZSTAN
       ALB.   GEORGIA AZERBAIJAN   TURKMENISTAN TAJIKISTAN   CHINA
TUNISIA   TURKEY ARMENIA   SOUTH
   MALTA   CYPRUS SYRIA   AFGHANISTAN   KOREA
MOROCCO   LEB. ─   IRAN
               ISRAEL ─   PAKISTAN
ALGERIA PALESTINE JORDAN   NEPAL BHUTAN
        AUTHORITY   BURMA LAOS
              EGYPT   QATAR UAE   INDIA BANGLADESH   THAILAND VIETNAM
CAPE   CAMBODIA PHILIPPINES
VERDE MAURITANIA MALI   ERITREA YEMEN   SRI LANKA
SENEGAL   NIGER CHAD SUDAN   DJIBOUTI   MALDIVES   MALAYSIA
AMBIA   BF   SINGAPORE
GUINEA CÔTE NIGERIA CENTRAL ETHIOPIA   INDONESIA
UINEA- D'IVOIRE GHANA   AFRICAN REP. UGANDA SOMALIA   EAST TIMOR
BISSAU   TOGO CAMEROON   KENYA
SIERRA LIBERIA BENIN EQUATORIAL DEM. REP. RWANDA
LEONE   GUINEA OF CONGO TANZANIA SEYCHELLES
          SAO TOME GABON BURUNDI
          & PRINCIPE CONGO   COMOROS
                  ANGOLA ZAMBIA MALAWI
                               ZIMBABWE MADAGASCAR MAURITIUS
                  NAMIBIA BOTSWANA   MOZAMBIQUE
                         SWAZILAND
                  SOUTH ─LESOTHO
                  AFRICA

AUSTRALIA

SOLOMON
ISLANDS   SAMOA
VANUATU   FIJI
          TONGA

PAPUA
NEW
GUINEA

Over half the residents of many cities live in slums, with limited or no access to adequate shelter, water and sanitation, or education and health services.

People's living conditions affect their physical, mental and social health. The increased morbidity and mortality resulting from overcrowding and poor sanitation that was demonstrated during the 19th-century industrial revolution in Europe remains an all-too-evident outcome of the rapid urbanization of developing countries and the increase in slum dwellings.

"Housing" includes not only a physical dwelling place, but the psychological and social aspects of the home, the immediate environment and the community. "Healthy housing" combines adequate shelter, space, privacy, security, safety, and basic infrastructure such as water and sanitation, with access to work, services and facilities – all of which contribute to a person's well-being.

In too many cases, however, housing fails to protect its occupants. Many dwellings are damp and mouldy, with air polluted by the particulates resulting from the burning of solid fuels, and by tobacco smoke, putting their occupants at increased risk of asthma and respiratory diseases. In cold climates, inadequate heating and insulation increase the risk of hypothermia, respiratory disease and heart disease. Residents of poor housing are also at risk of domestic injuries, including falls, fires, and poisoning.

There are clear health benefits for communities with affordable housing designed to promote physical activity and with access to health services.

DEVELOPMENT OF SLUMS

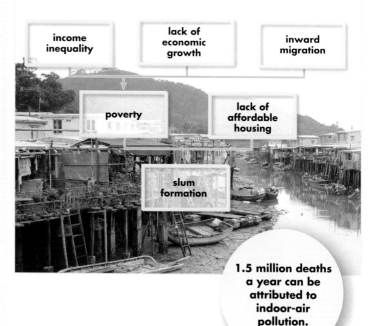

income inequality

lack of economic growth

inward migration

poverty

lack of affordable housing

slum formation

1.5 million deaths a year can be attributed to indoor-air pollution.

More than half the world's population use solid fuels for cooking.

74%

74%

77%

36%

18%

18%

SMOKY HOMES
Percentage of people using solid fuels for cooking
2005

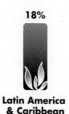

Latin America & Caribbean

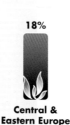

Central & Eastern Europe

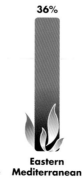

Eastern Mediterranean

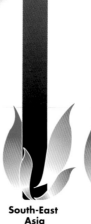

South-East Asia

Western Pacific

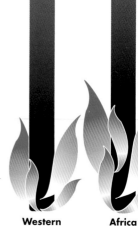

Africa

HOUSING CONDITIONS

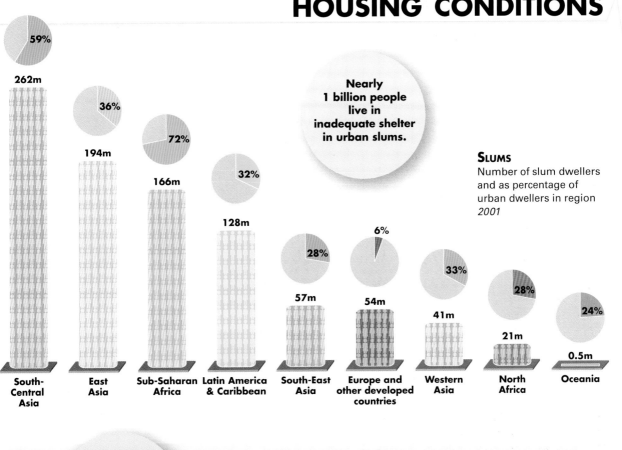

Nearly 1 billion people live in inadequate shelter in urban slums.

SLUMS
Number of slum dwellers and as percentage of urban dwellers in region
2001

59%
262m
South-Central Asia

36%
194m
East Asia

72%
166m
Sub-Saharan Africa

32%
128m
Latin America & Caribbean

28%
57m
South-East Asia

6%
54m
Europe and other developed countries

33%
41m
Western Asia

28%
21m
North Africa

24%
0.5m
Oceania

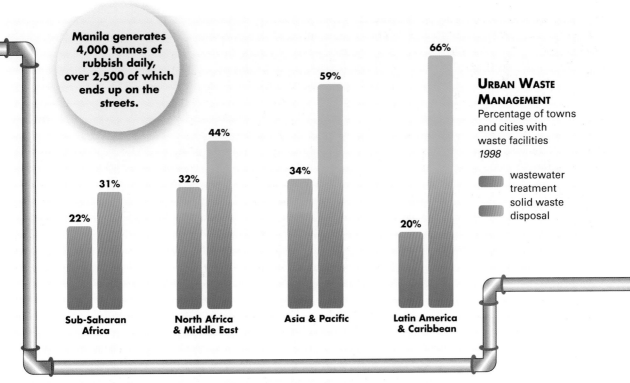

Manila generates 4,000 tonnes of rubbish daily, over 2,500 of which ends up on the streets.

URBAN WASTE MANAGEMENT
Percentage of towns and cities with waste facilities
1998

wastewater treatment

solid waste disposal

22%
31%
Sub-Saharan Africa

32%
44%
North Africa & Middle East

34%
59%
Asia & Pacific

20%
66%
Latin America & Caribbean

Employment and working conditions influence health and social position.

Work gives people money, status and social approval, which influence physical, mental and social health. Employment in developing countries is predominantly in the agricultural sector, with industry and services dominating in wealthier countries. Globally, women are more likely to be employed on an informal basis.

Unemployed people and their families are at higher risk of ill-health and of premature death. Ill-health also puts people at risk of unemployment and financial problems, including debt. Unemployment and unsatisfactory or insecure jobs can cause stress, anxiety, depression, and are risk factors for heart disease and other serious chronic illnesses. Parental unemployment and childhood poverty may have life-long effects on health.

Work can be dangerous. It can expose employees to risk of injury, illness or death. People employed in high-demand, low-control jobs have poorer health than those with more control over their work.

Although the number of children working worldwide has declined recently, 20 percent of those aged five to 17 are estimated to be economically active: 14 percent (218 million) work illegally, and 8 percent (126 million) are engaged in hazardous work.

Young people aged 15 to 24 make up nearly half the world's jobless, although they are only 25 percent of the working-age population.

UNEMPLOYMENT
Percentage of working-age people who are unemployed
latest available 1994–2004

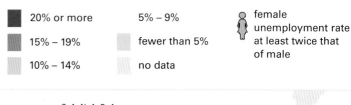

- 20% or more
- 15% – 19%
- 10% – 14%
- 5% – 9%
- fewer than 5%
- no data

female unemployment rate at least twice that of male

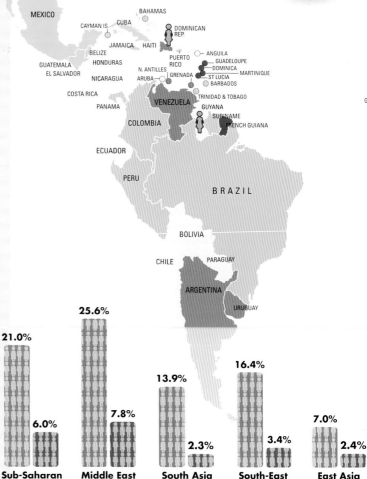

Over one-fifth of the global workforce works more than 48 hours a week.

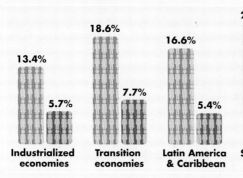

13.4% / 5.7%	18.6% / 7.7%	16.6% / 5.4%	21.0% / 6.0%	25.6% / 7.8%	13.9% / 2.3%	16.4% / 3.4%	7.0% / 2.4%
Industrialized economies	Transition economies	Latin America & Caribbean	Sub-Saharan Africa	Middle East & North Africa	South Asia	South-East Asia	East Asia

WORKING CONDITIONS

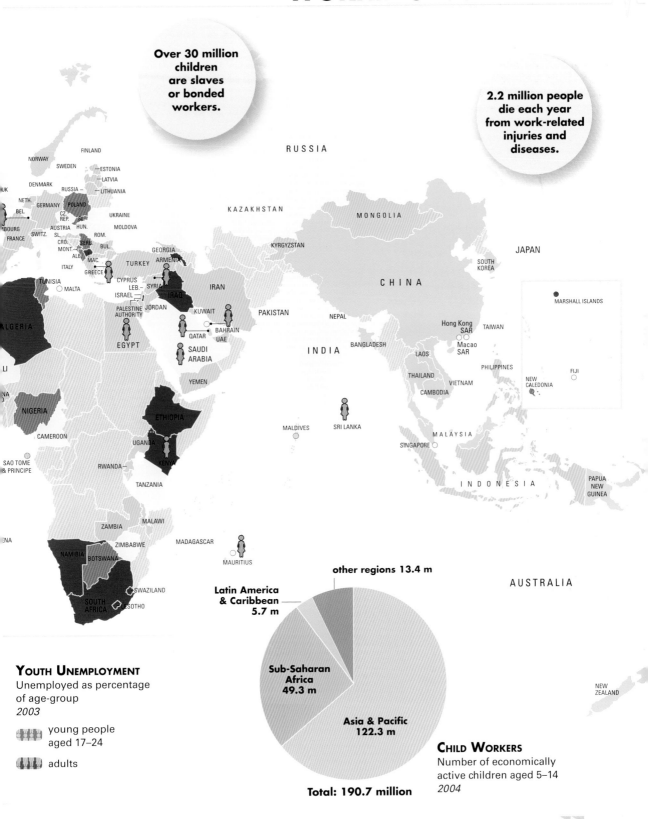

Over 30 million children are slaves or bonded workers.

2.2 million people die each year from work-related injuries and diseases.

FINLAND
NORWAY
SWEDEN
ESTONIA
LATVIA
DENMARK
LITHUANIA
UK
NETH.
GERMANY
POLAND
RUSSIA
BEL.
CZ. REP.
UKRAINE
MBOURG
AUSTRIA
HUN.
MOLDOVA
FRANCE
SWITZ.
SL.
CRO.
ROM.
MONT.
SERB.
ALB.
BUL.
ITALY
MAC.
GEORGIA
GREECE
TURKEY
ARMENIA
TUNISIA
MALTA
CYPRUS
LEB.
SYRIA
IRAQ
IRAN
ISRAEL
JORDAN
ALGERIA
PALESTINE AUTHORITY
KUWAIT
BAHRAIN
QATAR
UAE
EGYPT
SAUDI ARABIA
YEMEN

RUSSIA
KAZAKHSTAN
MONGOLIA
JAPAN
KYRGYZSTAN
SOUTH KOREA
CHINA
PAKISTAN
NEPAL
Hong Kong SAR
TAIWAN
INDIA
BANGLADESH
Macao SAR
LAOS
PHILIPPINES
THAILAND
VIETNAM
CAMBODIA
MARSHALL ISLANDS
NEW CALEDONIA
FIJI

MALI
NIGERIA
CAMEROON
ETHIOPIA
SAO TOME & PRINCIPE
UGANDA
RWANDA
KENYA
TANZANIA

MALDIVES
SRI LANKA
MALAYSIA
SINGAPORE
INDONESIA
PAPUA NEW GUINEA

ZAMBIA
MALAWI
MADAGASCAR
NAMIBIA
ZIMBABWE
BOTSWANA
MAURITIUS
SWAZILAND
SOUTH AFRICA
LESOTHO

AUSTRALIA

NEW ZEALAND

YOUTH UNEMPLOYMENT
Unemployed as percentage of age-group
2003

young people aged 17–24

adults

other regions 13.4 m

Latin America & Caribbean 5.7 m

Sub-Saharan Africa 49.3 m

Asia & Pacific 122.3 m

Total: 190.7 million

CHILD WORKERS
Number of economically active children aged 5–14
2004

Injury 54–55; Human Resources 88–89

Low government spending on healthcare is a major obstacle to improving health.

The average government spending on health in the least-developed countries falls well below the $34 per person per year estimated as the minimum required to provide essential healthcare.

Public spending on health comes from a range of sources, including government money, loans, aid and grants from international agencies and non-governmental organizations, and social insurance funds. It reduces the necessity for private spending – payments made for healthcare directly by individuals or organizations – but health-sector reforms in many countries are increasingly requiring healthcare users to pay fees even in the public sector.

There are wide disparities between countries in the level of government spending on healthcare, but within countries there are also huge disparities in the use of publicly funded primary healthcare services between rich and poor. Where there are user fees, access to healthcare services is related to ability to pay. Fees clearly deter poor people from seeking healthcare.

There is a well-recognized need to reorient health spending and health services towards primary healthcare, and to activities that prevent illness and promote health. Investment is needed to improve the effectiveness of existing healthcare-delivery systems and in monitoring outcomes. The Primary Health Care approach, described in the Alma Ata Declaration on Health in 1978, promotes a multi-sectoral approach to the determinants of health, integration of services, equality of access and use, appropriate health technology and community involvement in the healthcare system.

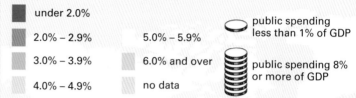

PUBLIC EXPENDITURE

Share of GDP spent on healthcare
2003

- under 2.0%
- 2.0% – 2.9%
- 3.0% – 3.9%
- 4.0% – 4.9%
- 5.0% – 5.9%
- 6.0% and over
- no data

public spending less than 1% of GDP

public spending 8% or more of GDP

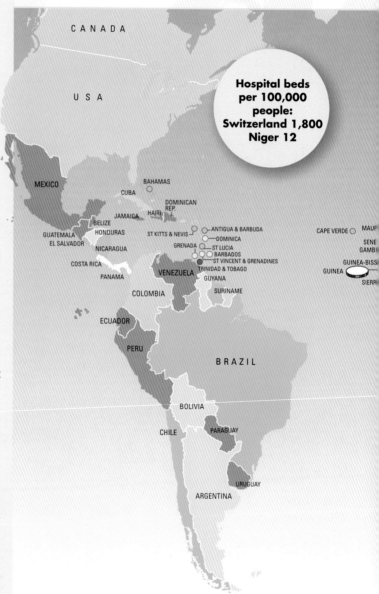

Hospital beds per 100,000 people: Switzerland 1,800 Niger 12

CANADA

USA

MEXICO

BAHAMAS

CUBA

DOMINICAN REP.

JAMAICA

HAITI

BELIZE

GUATEMALA

HONDURAS

EL SALVADOR

NICARAGUA

COSTA RICA

PANAMA

ST KITTS & NEVIS

ANTIGUA & BARBUDA

DOMINICA

GRENADA

ST LUCIA

BARBADOS

ST VINCENT & GRENADINES

TRINIDAD & TOBAGO

VENEZUELA

GUYANA

COLOMBIA

SURINAME

ECUADOR

PERU

BRAZIL

BOLIVIA

CHILE

PARAGUAY

URUGUAY

ARGENTINA

CAPE VERDE

MAU[F]

SENE

GAMB[I]

GUINEA-BISS[A]

GUINEA

SIERR[A]

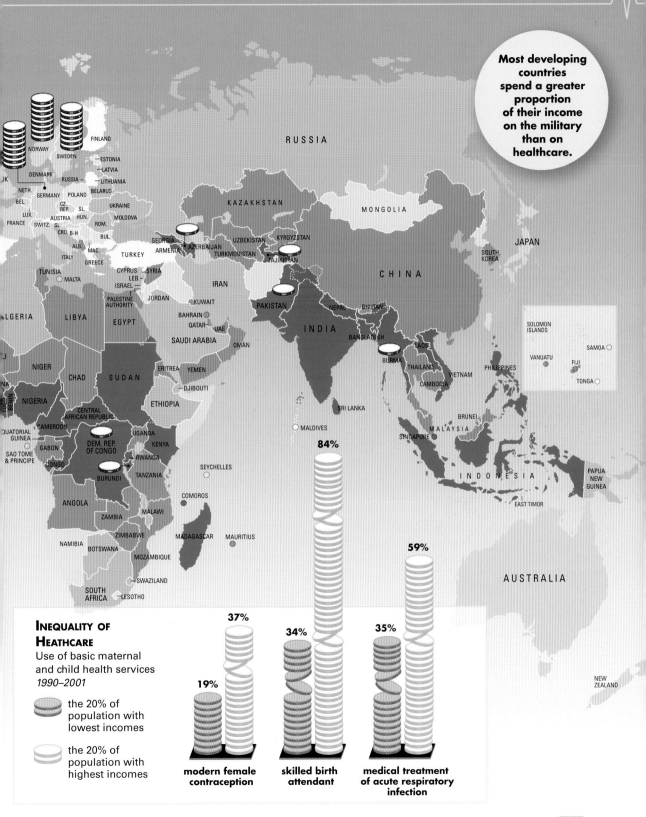

Most developing
countries
spend a greater
proportion
of their income
on the military
than on
healthcare.

RUSSIA

FINLAND

NORWAY
SWEDEN
DENMARK
RUSSIA
ESTONIA
LATVIA
LITHUANIA
BELARUS
NETH.
BEL.
LUX.
FRANCE
GERMANY
CZ.
REP.
AUSTRIA
SWITZ. SL.
POLAND
SL.
HUN.
ROM.
MOLDOVA
UKRAINE
CRO. B-H
ALB.
MAC
BUL.
ITALY
GREECE
TUNISIA
MALTA
TURKEY
CYPRUS
LEB.
ISRAEL
SYRIA
JORDAN

KAZAKHSTAN
MONGOLIA
JAPAN

GEORGIA
ARMENIA
AZERBAIJAN
UZBEKISTAN
KYRGYZSTAN
TURKMENISTAN
TAJIKISTAN
CHINA
SOUTH
KOREA

IRAN
KUWAIT

LGERIA
LIBYA
EGYPT
SAUDI ARABIA
OMAN
PALESTINE
AUTHORITY
BAHRAIN
QATAR
UAE
PAKISTAN
NEPAL
BHUTAN
INDIA
BANGLADESH

SOLOMON
ISLANDS

NIGER
CHAD
SUDAN
ERITREA
YEMEN
DJIBOUTI
BURMA
LAOS
THAILAND
VIETNAM
CAMBODIA
PHILIPPINES

VANUATU
FIJI
SAMOA
TONGA

NIGERIA
ETHIOPIA
SRI LANKA
BRUNEI
MALAYSIA
SINGAPORE

QUATORIAL
GUINEA
CENTRAL
AFRICAN REPUBLIC
CAMEROON
UGANDA
KENYA
MALDIVES
INDONESIA
PAPUA
NEW
GUINEA

SAO TOME
& PRINCIPE
GABON
ONGO
DEM. REP.
OF CONGO
RWANDA
BURUNDI
TANZANIA
SEYCHELLES
EAST TIMOR

ANGOLA
COMOROS
ZAMBIA
MALAWI
MADAGASCAR
MAURITIUS

NAMIBIA
ZIMBABWE
BOTSWANA
MOZAMBIQUE
AUSTRALIA

SWAZILAND
SOUTH
AFRICA
LESOTHO

84%

59%

NEW
ZEALAND

INEQUALITY OF HEATHCARE

Use of basic maternal
and child health services
1990–2001

the 20% of
population with
lowest incomes

the 20% of
population with
highest incomes

37%

19%

modern female
contraception

34%

skilled birth
attendant

35%

medical treatment
of acute respiratory
infection

Tobacco use is the major preventable risk factor for cancer and heart disease.

Tobacco is highly addictive. Tobacco smoke contains over 4,000 chemicals, at least 60 of which can cause cancer. Smokers have an increased risk of developing cancer – especially lung cancer – heart disease, stroke, lung and many other diseases. Smoking in pregnancy damages the foetus and has long-term effects after birth.

Passive smoking – exposure to environmental tobacco smoke, which has higher levels of gaseous carcinogens and smaller-sized particulate matter than inhaled smoke – also increases these health risks in non-smokers. Children exposed to adult's smoke are at risk of respiratory disease and possibly of cancer and heart disease in later life. The prevalence of smoking in women is increasing, with consequent increases in the prevalence of tobacco-related disease and deaths in women.

Daily smoking is most prevalent among the lowest-income households in all regions except Europe. Among the poorest households, up to 10 percent of household expenditure is on tobacco. Smokers and their families lose income through illness. High rates of tobacco use in countries with the poorest health resources will increase global health inequalities.

Policy responses include banning smoking in workplaces, banning advertising, support for smokers who want to quit, and increasing the price. The WHO Framework Convention on Tobacco Control, adopted in 2003, requires countries to impose restrictions on tobacco advertising, sponsorship and promotion, establish new packaging and labelling of tobacco products, establish clean indoor-air controls, and strengthen legislation to clamp down on tobacco smuggling.

CANCER DEATHS CAUSED BY SMOKING
Percentage by site of cancer
2005 or most recent estimate

- 71% trachea, bronchus, lung
- 59% larynx
- 39% upper aerodigestive
- 27% bladder
- 26% kidney
- 21% pancreas
- 12% leukaemia
- 12% liver
- 11% stomach
- 3% cervix
- 17% all cancers

Lung-cancer deaths in women are increasing more than in men in some countries.

- 520m If present smoking patterns continue
- 500m If youth uptake halves by 2020
- 340m If adult consumption halves by 2020
- 220m
- 190m
- 70m

2000   2025   2050

TOBACCO DEATH OUTLOOK
Effect of smoking patterns on cumulative tobacco deaths
1950, projected to 2050
millions

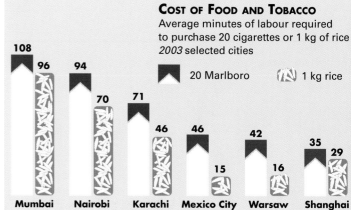

COST OF FOOD AND TOBACCO
Average minutes of labour required to purchase 20 cigarettes or 1 kg of rice
2003 selected cities

- 20 Marlboro
- 1 kg rice

City	20 Marlboro	1 kg rice
Mumbai, India	108	96
Nairobi, Kenya	94	70
Karachi, Pakistan	71	46
Mexico City, Mexico	46	15
Warsaw, Poland	42	16
Shanghai, China	35	29

Poverty 24–25; Housing Conditions 32–33; Working Conditions 34–35

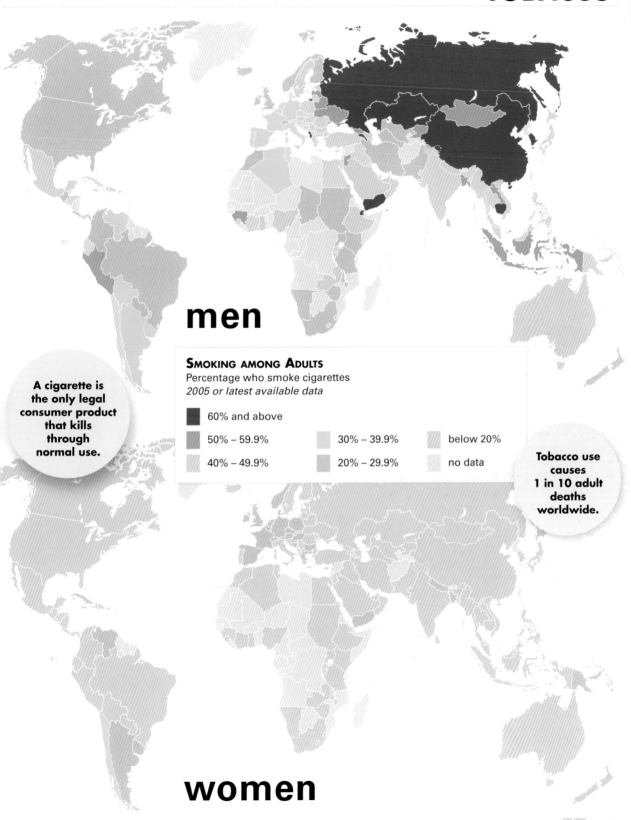

men

A cigarette is the only legal consumer product that kills through normal use.

SMOKING AMONG ADULTS
Percentage who smoke cigarettes
2005 or latest available data

- 60% and above
- 50% – 59.9%
- 40% – 49.9%
- 30% – 39.9%
- 20% – 29.9%
- below 20%
- no data

Tobacco use causes 1 in 10 adult deaths worldwide.

women

Addiction to alcohol and drugs causes major health problems for individuals and society.

Moderate amounts of alcohol may have some beneficial effects on health, but excessive alcohol consumption can have severe adverse effects on physical and mental health, and is a major cause of social harm. Alcohol consumption is both a risk factor and a protective factor for cardiovascular disease and stroke and is related to a range of cancers, mental disorders and other chronic diseases. In pregnancy, it may harm the foetus and have long-term consequences.

Alcohol consumption and binge drinking in young people are increasing in many countries. Alcohol use is associated with high-risk behaviours, including unsafe sex and use of other psychoactive substances, and is a major risk factor for road deaths and injuries, interpersonal injuries and assaults.

About five percent of people aged between 15 and 64 are estimated to use illicit drugs each year, although official figures are lower than this. No-one knows the true extent of illegal drug use as it is, by definition, hidden in the population. Estimates of prevalence are based on a combination of population surveys, data on drug seizures and drug-related crime, health-service data and drug-related deaths.

The price of opiates and cocaine is declining, while demand for treatment for drug-related problems is increasing in many countries. Heroin users commonly inject, and sharing needles increases the risk of HIV and hepatitis. Illegal drug use is closely linked to crime; problem drug users tend to be from the poorest sections of society.

ALCOHOL AND DRUG USE

Average litres of pure alcohol consumed per person
2003

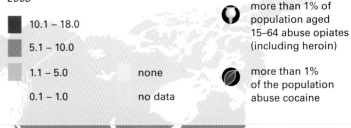

10.1 – 18.0		
5.1 – 10.0		
1.1 – 5.0	none	
0.1 – 1.0	no data	

more than 1% of population aged 15–64 abuse opiates (including heroin)

more than 1% of the population abuse cocaine

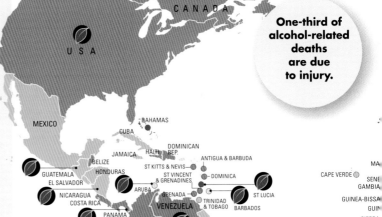

One-third of alcohol-related deaths are due to injury.

ILLEGAL DRUG USE

Regional breakdown
2005

- Africa
- Asia
- Europe
- North America
- Oceania
- South America

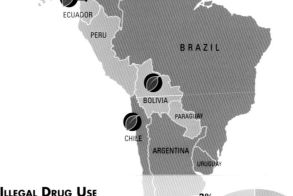

3% 8% 8%

15%

11%

55%

ecstasy

Poverty 24–25; Tobacco 38–39

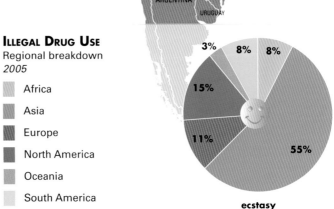

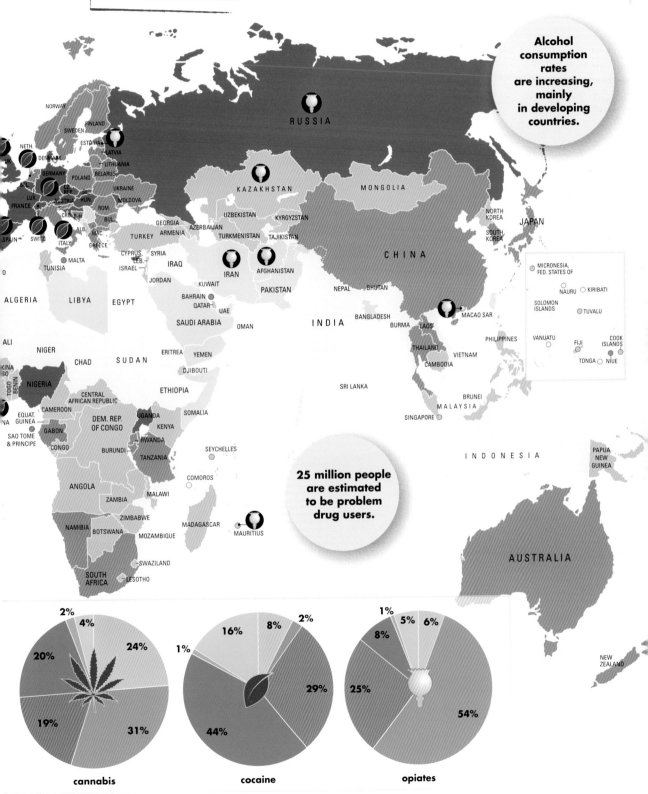

ALCOHOL AND DRUGS

Alcohol consumption rates are increasing, mainly in developing countries.

25 million people are estimated to be problem drug users.

NORWAY
SWEDEN
FINLAND
NETH.
DENMARK
ESTONIA
LATVIA
LITHUANIA
UK
GERMANY
POLAND
BELARUS
LUX.
CZ REP.
SK
FRANCE
AUSTRIA
HUN.
MOLDOVA
UKRAINE
SL
CRO B-H
ROM.
SPAIN
SWITZ.
ITALY
ALB.
BUL.
MAC.
GREECE
RUSSIA
KAZAKHSTAN
MONGOLIA
NORTH KOREA
JAPAN
SOUTH KOREA
GEORGIA
AZERBAIJAN
ARMENIA
TURKEY
UZBEKISTAN
KYRGYZSTAN
TURKMENISTAN
TAJIKISTAN
CHINA
MALTA
TUNISIA
CYPRUS
LEB.
SYRIA
ISRAEL
IRAQ
JORDAN
IRAN
AFGHANISTAN
PAKISTAN
NEPAL
BHUTAN
MACAO SAR
ALGERIA
LIBYA
EGYPT
KUWAIT
BAHRAIN
QATAR
UAE
SAUDI ARABIA
OMAN
INDIA
BANGLADESH
BURMA
LAOS
PHILIPPINES
ALI
NIGER
CHAD
SUDAN
ERITREA
YEMEN
THAILAND
VIETNAM
CAMBODIA
KINA SO
NIGERIA
CENTRAL AFRICAN REPUBLIC
ETHIOPIA
DJIBOUTI
SOMALIA
SRI LANKA
BRUNEI
MALAYSIA
TOGO
BENIN
CAMEROON
UGANDA
KENYA
SINGAPORE
EQUAT. GUINEA
NA
GABON
DEM. REP. OF CONGO
RWANDA
SAO TOME & PRINCIPE
CONGO
BURUNDI
TANZANIA
SEYCHELLES
COMOROS
INDONESIA
PAPUA NEW GUINEA
ANGOLA
ZAMBIA
MALAWI
MADAGASCAR
MAURITIUS
NAMIBIA
ZIMBABWE
BOTSWANA
MOZAMBIQUE
SWAZILAND
SOUTH AFRICA
LESOTHO
AUSTRALIA
NEW ZEALAND

MICRONESIA, FED. STATES OF
NAURU
KIRIBATI
SOLOMON ISLANDS
TUVALU
VANUATU
FIJI
COOK ISLANDS
TONGA
NIUE

cannabis

2%
4%
24%
20%
19%
31%

cocaine

16%
8%
2%
1%
29%
44%

opiates

1%
5%
6%
8%
25%
54%

Major Causes of Death

As percentage of all deaths
estimates for 2002

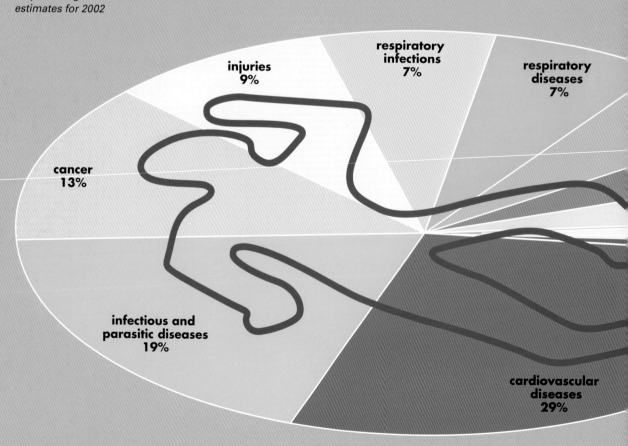

injuries
9%

respiratory
infections
7%

respiratory
diseases
7%

cancer
13%

infectious and
parasitic diseases
19%

cardiovascular
diseases
29%

PART 3 〜

HEALTH PROBLEMS

Over the last century there has been an enormous change in patterns of disease and death. The combination of unhealthy diets, physical inactivity and smoking are major risk factors for cardiovascular disease and cancers, the leading non-communicable diseases. Already responsible for over 40 percent of all deaths, they are likely to increase their toll as the century progresses. Deaths and disability from injuries and violence are also increasing.

Most of the premature deaths caused by communicable diseases occur in Sub-Saharan Africa. More than half of the deaths of children aged under five result from them contracting communicable diseases, many of which could have been prevented by immunization.

Because the quality of health statistics varies, countries with good health information systems may appear to have more severe problems than countries with limited or no data. And what even the best data may hide is that within most countries there are disparities between the health of the poorest and the wealthiest sections of society.

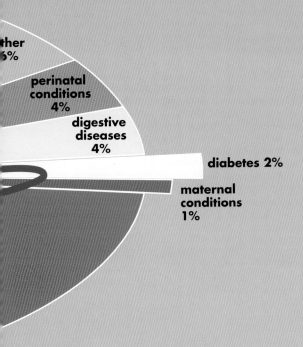

ther
6%

perinatal
conditions
4%

digestive
diseases
4%

diabetes 2%

maternal
conditions
1%

Cancers are projected to be the leading single cause of death worldwide by 2010.

"Cancer" refers to over 100 different diseases, affecting all parts of the body. Many cancers can now be prevented and cured: there have been dramatic advances in treatments in recent years. Death rates for many common cancers are decreasing in developed countries, but the prevalence and incidence of cancers is increasing in poorer countries, where resources to manage cancer are limited.

At least one-third of all cancers are preventable. Cancers could be prevented by modifying the major risk factors: tobacco, diet, physical inactivity, infection, radiation, and occupational exposures. About one in four cancers in developing countries is caused by infection. Cervical cancer is related to infection with human papilloma virus (HPV), and hepatitis B (HBV) and C viruses cause liver cancer. Vaccines are available to prevent HPV and HBV.

Screening tests exist for several major cancers. Early detection can help reduce cancer mortality where there is prompt effective treatment. Screening programmes for breast and cervical cancer have led to declines in invasive disease and deaths.

Cancer registries collect, analyze and interpret data on cancer for a population, providing essential information for planning and evaluating cancer-control programmes.

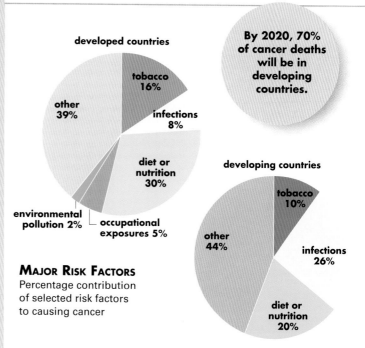

developed countries

By 2020, 70% of cancer deaths will be in developing countries.

tobacco 16%
infections 8%
other 39%
diet or nutrition 30%
environmental pollution 2%
occupational exposures 5%

developing countries

tobacco 10%
other 44%
infections 26%
diet or nutrition 20%

MAJOR RISK FACTORS
Percentage contribution of selected risk factors to causing cancer

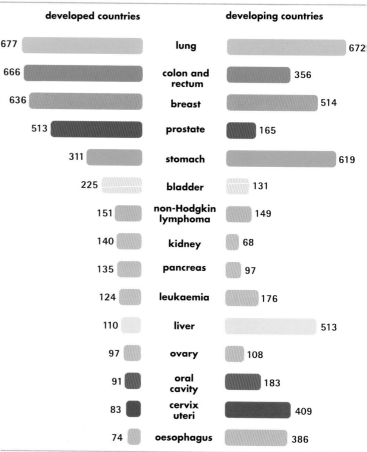

developed countries		developing countries
677	lung	672
666	colon and rectum	356
636	breast	514
513	prostate	165
311	stomach	619
225	bladder	131
151	non-Hodgkin lymphoma	149
140	kidney	68
135	pancreas	97
124	leukaemia	176
110	liver	513
97	ovary	108
91	oral cavity	183
83	cervix uteri	409
74	oesophagus	386

GLOBAL DIFFERENCES
Number of new cancer cases in developed and developing countries
2002
thousands

Food and Nutrition 28–29; Healthcare 36–37; Tobacco 38–39

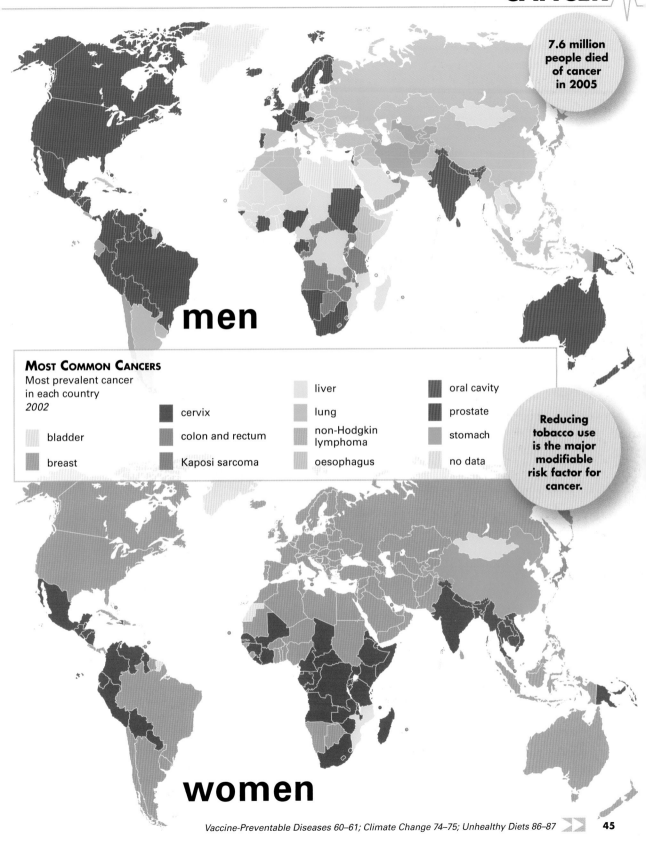

7.6 million people died of cancer in 2005

men

MOST COMMON CANCERS

Most prevalent cancer in each country
2002

- bladder
- breast
- cervix
- colon and rectum
- Kaposi sarcoma
- liver
- lung
- non-Hodgkin lymphoma
- oesophagus
- oral cavity
- prostate
- stomach
- no data

Reducing tobacco use is the major modifiable risk factor for cancer.

women

Heart disease and stroke are, together, the leading cause of adult death worldwide.

Cardiovascular disease (CVD) includes coronary heart disease (disease of the blood vessels of the heart), cerebrovascular disease (disease of blood vessels of the brain), high blood pressure, heart failure and rheumatic heart disease. Heart attacks and strokes are caused mainly by blockages of blood vessels to parts of the heart or brain.

Although the risk of CVD increases markedly after the age of 40, the risk factors for developing the disease start in early life. Many deaths could be prevented by improvements in: tobacco use, diet, physical activity, obesity, blood pressure and cholesterol. High intakes of salt increase blood pressure, and some saturated animal fats and transfats increase cholesterol. Obesity and type 2 diabetes increase the risk of CVD. In most countries it is poorer people who have more risk factors, and suffer higher levels of disease.

While rates of disease and death are decreasing in many developed countries as result of better prevention and control of blood pressure and cholesterol, they are increasing in many developing countries as a result of improved life expectancy, urbanization and changes in lifestyle risk factors, such as tobacco use and consumption of animal fats.

Screening for high blood pressure and raised cholesterol can detect risk factors before symptoms develop and allow for interventions to prevent progression.

CARDIOVASCULAR DISEASE DEATHS
Age-standardized mortality rate
per 100,000 people
2002

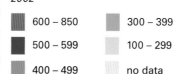

- 600 – 850
- 500 – 599
- 400 – 499
- 300 – 399
- 100 – 299
- no data

🌡 age-standardized mortality rate for stroke of over 175 per 100,000 *2002*

Age-standardized rates enable a comparison to be made between populations with different age structures.

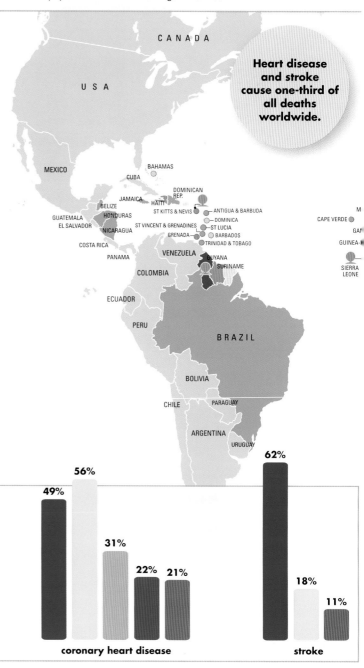

Heart disease and stroke cause one-third of all deaths worldwide.

MAJOR RISK FACTORS
Percentage contribution of selected risk factors to coronary heart disease and stroke
2002

- suboptimal systolic blood pressure
- high cholesterol
- low fruit and vegetable intake
- physical inactivity
- obesity

coronary heart disease
49% 56% 31% 22% 21%

stroke
62% 18% 11%

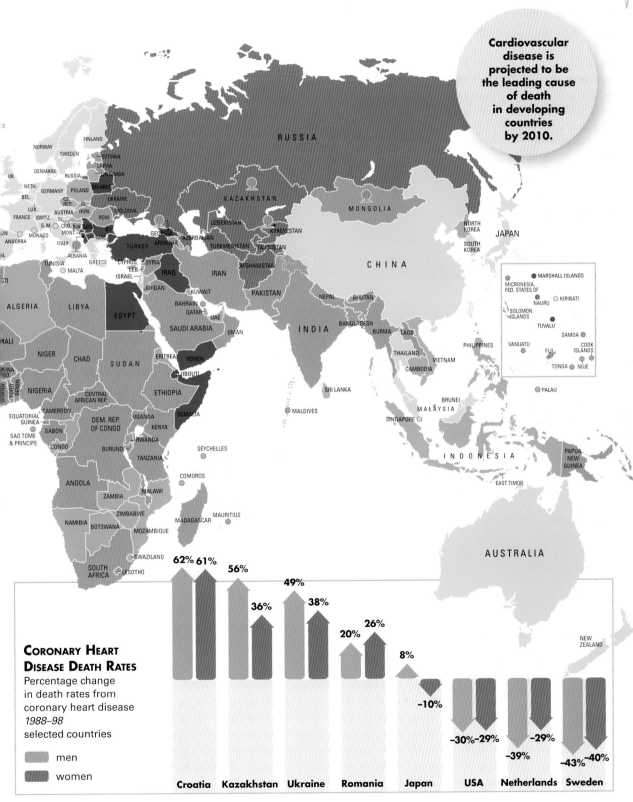

Cardiovascular disease is projected to be the leading cause of death in developing countries by 2010.

CORONARY HEART DISEASE DEATH RATES
Percentage change in death rates from coronary heart disease *1988–98* selected countries

men

women

62% 61%   56%   49%   20%   8%

36%   38%   26%   -10%

-30% -29%   -39%   -43% -40%

-29%

Croatia   Kazakhstan   Ukraine   Romania   Japan   USA   Netherlands   Sweden

246 million people have diabetes, 80 percent of whom live in developing countries.

Diabetes mellitus is a chronic, potentially debilitating disease that can kill. Insulin is a hormone that brings sugar from the blood to the body's cells to be used for energy. In diabetes blood-sugar levels are high, either because the body cannot produce enough insulin (type 1 diabetes), or because it cannot use the insulin it does produce effectively (type 2 diabetes).

Chronic high blood-sugar can damage the heart and blood vessels, kidneys, nerves, and eyes, and cause disability and death from heart disease, stroke, kidney failure, amputations and blindness.

It is not yet possible to prevent type 1 diabetes, and people with the condition need to take insulin to lower their blood-sugar. However, more than 90 percent of people with diabetes have type 2, which is related to excess calorie intake, obesity and a sedentary lifestyle. Onset can be prevented, and the impact can be reduced by changes in diet and physical activity. Non-insulin drugs may be used, and insulin is not usually needed.

Until recently, type 2 diabetes was considered a disease of older people, but an increasing number of children and young people are being affected.

Complications of diabetes can be prevented by appropriate care, treatment and monitoring. Access to life-saving treatments, education and care that delay or prevent complications are essential.

DIABETES MELLITUS
Percentage of population with condition
2003

■ 10.0% or more	▨ 2.5% – 4.9%
7.5% – 9.9%	fewer than 2.5%
5.0% – 7.4%	no data

20% or more of adult population obese (Body Mass Index more than 30)
latest available data 1995–2005

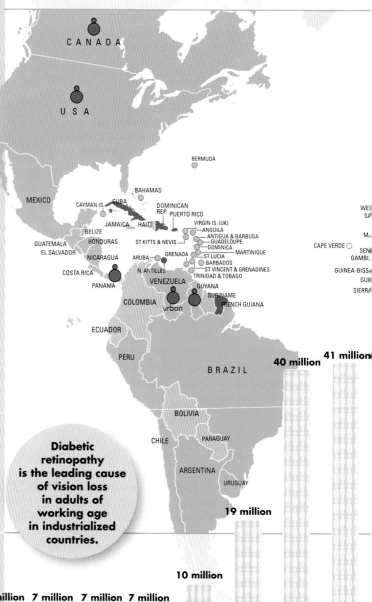

Diabetic retinopathy is the leading cause of vision loss in adults of working age in industrialized countries.

TOP TEN
Largest populations of people aged over 19 with diabetes
2007

Egypt	Mexico	Pakistan	Japan	Germany	Brazil	Russia	USA	China	India
4 million	6 million	7 million	7 million	7 million	7 million	10 million	19 million	40 million	41 million

Heart Disease and Stroke 46–47

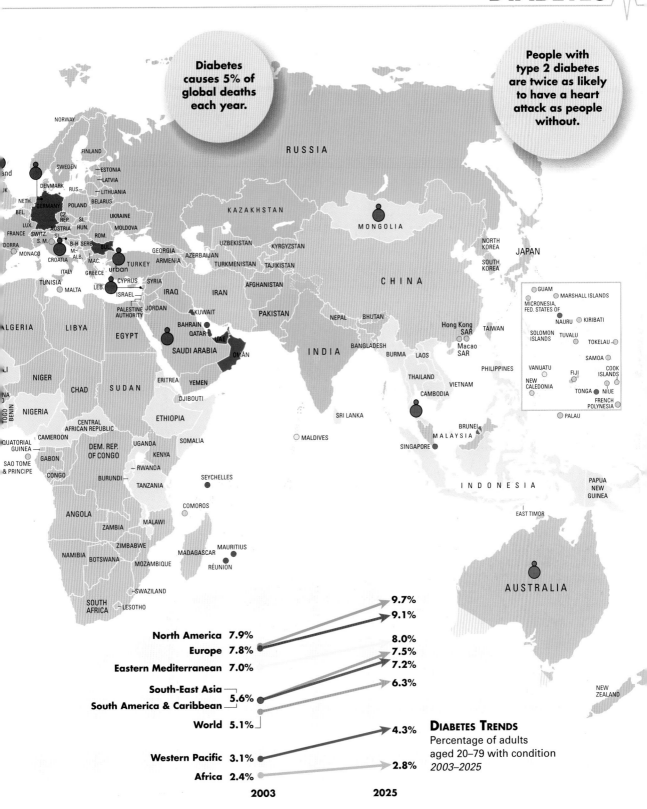

Diabetes causes 5% of global deaths each year.

People with type 2 diabetes are twice as likely to have a heart attack as people without.

NORWAY
FINLAND
SWEDEN
ESTONIA
LATVIA
DENMARK
LITHUANIA
RUS.
BELARUS
NETH.
GERMANY
POLAND
BEL
CZ. REP.
UKRAINE
LUX.
AUSTRIA
SL.
HUN.
MOLDOVA
FRANCE
SWITZ.
ROM.
S. M.
SL.
DORRA
B-H
SERB.
BUL.
MONACO
M-
ALB.
GEORGIA
CROATIA
MAC.
TURKEY
ARMENIA
AZERBAIJAN
ITALY
GREECE
urban
TUNISIA
CYPRUS
SYRIA
MALTA
LEB.
IRAQ
IRAN
ISRAEL
PALESTINE AUTHORITY
JORDAN
ALGERIA
LIBYA
KUWAIT
EGYPT
BAHRAIN
QATAR
UAE
SAUDI ARABIA
OMAN
NIGER
CHAD
SUDAN
ERITREA
YEMEN
NIGERIA
DJIBOUTI
ETHIOPIA
TOGO
BENIN
CAMEROON
CENTRAL AFRICAN REPUBLIC
UGANDA
SOMALIA
EQUATORIAL GUINEA
GABON
DEM. REP. OF CONGO
KENYA
SAO TOME & PRINCIPE
CONGO
RWANDA
BURUNDI
TANZANIA
SEYCHELLES
ANGOLA
COMOROS
ZAMBIA
MALAWI
ZIMBABWE
MADAGASCAR
MAURITIUS
NAMIBIA
BOTSWANA
MOZAMBIQUE
RÉUNION
SWAZILAND
SOUTH AFRICA
LESOTHO

RUSSIA
KAZAKHSTAN
MONGOLIA
NORTH KOREA
JAPAN
SOUTH KOREA
UZBEKISTAN
KYRGYZSTAN
TURKMENISTAN
TAJIKISTAN
CHINA
AFGHANISTAN
PAKISTAN
NEPAL
BHUTAN
Hong Kong SAR
TAIWAN
BANGLADESH
Macao SAR
INDIA
BURMA
LAOS
PHILIPPINES
THAILAND
VIETNAM
CAMBODIA
SRI LANKA
MALDIVES
BRUNEI
MALAYSIA
SINGAPORE
INDONESIA
PAPUA NEW GUINEA
EAST TIMOR
AUSTRALIA
NEW ZEALAND

GUAM
MARSHALL ISLANDS
MICRONESIA, FED. STATES OF
NAURU
KIRIBATI
SOLOMON ISLANDS
TUVALU
TOKELAU
SAMOA
VANUATU
FIJI
COOK ISLANDS
NEW CALEDONIA
TONGA
NIUE
FRENCH POLYNESIA
PALAU

North America 7.9% → 9.7%
Europe 7.8% → 9.1%
Eastern Mediterranean 7.0% → 8.0%
→ 7.5%
→ 7.2%
South-East Asia → 6.3%
South America & Caribbean 5.6%
World 5.1%
→ 4.3%
Western Pacific 3.1%
Africa 2.4% → 2.8%
2003   2025

DIABETES TRENDS
Percentage of adults
aged 20–79 with condition
2003–2025

One person in four is likely to develop a mental or behavioural disorder at some time.

Mental health is essential to health. Five of the ten leading causes of disability and premature death worldwide are psychiatric conditions. Nearly 900,000 people die by suicide each year.

Mental health and illness have multiple social, psychological and biological determinants. Everyone is at risk of mental illness, but for the poor and disadvantaged people in every country, this risk is increased.

Mental health and physical health and illness are closely linked. Mental illness can be caused by, and be an effect of, cancer, heart disease, diabetes, and infectious diseases such as HIV/AIDS. Without treatment it can cause unhealthy behaviours, poor compliance with prescribed treatments, and a lower chance of recovery from physical illness.

The seriousness of mental illness is poorly recognized. For most disorders there are treatments that would enable sufferers to function effectively, but these are often unavailable. Few middle- or low-income countries spend more than 1 percent of their health budget on mental health. Investment is needed in appropriate training for workers in primary healthcare, mental health specialists and community-based care facilities, and in improving coverage for the poorest.

Prevention and effective mental-health promotion requires linkages across public sectors, including health, education, employment, housing, environment, criminal justice and human rights.

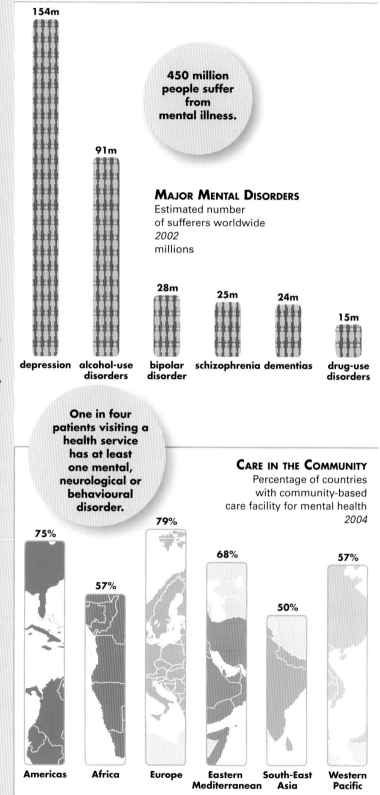

450 million people suffer from mental illness.

MAJOR MENTAL DISORDERS
Estimated number of sufferers worldwide
2002
millions

depression	alcohol-use disorders	bipolar disorder	schizophrenia	dementias	drug-use disorders
154m	91m	28m	25m	24m	15m

One in four patients visiting a health service has at least one mental, neurological or behavioural disorder.

CARE IN THE COMMUNITY
Percentage of countries with community-based care facility for mental health
2004

Americas	Africa	Europe	Eastern Mediterranean	South-East Asia	Western Pacific
75%	57%	79%	68%	50%	57%

Tobacco 38–39; Alcohol and Drugs 40–41

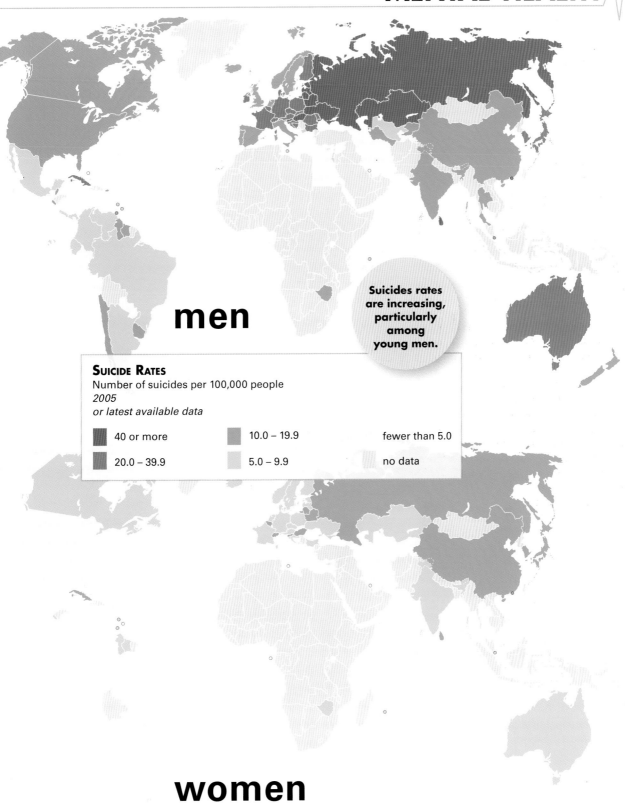

men

Suicides rates are increasing, particularly among young men.

SUICIDE RATES
Number of suicides per 100,000 people
2005
or latest available data

40 or more	10.0 – 19.9	fewer than 5.0
20.0 – 39.9	5.0 – 9.9	no data

women

Interpersonal violence kills, and can have long-lasting health effects on survivors.

Violent acts can be physical, psychological, sexual, or involve deprivation or neglect. Interpersonal violence includes violence or neglect towards children by parents or carers, towards older people and intimate partners. It includes assaults by strangers, and other intentional uses of force or power likely to result in injury, death, psychological harm, mal-development or deprivation. The damaging health effects of violence may last for many years after the initial abuse, or be permanent. Collective violence between groups and nations result in deaths, injury and displacement.

Measuring violence, especially non-fatal violence, is very difficult, and needs to be improved. Violent deaths – in particular those of children, women and older people – are sometimes concealed as accidents or as due to natural causes, especially where such deaths are not routinely investigated. Most women who are murdered are killed by their intimate partners. Many violent acts are not reported or recorded, especially intimate-partner violence against women, rapes and female infanticide.

All social groups experience violence, but the poor are consistently shown to be at greatest risk. Violence is often predictable and preventable. Prevention strategies need to bring together many disciplines and sectors to address the underlying causes of violence in individuals, families, close relationships, communities, and society as a whole.

One form of violence against children that has strong social and cultural roots is female genital mutilation/cutting (often called female circumcision), which involves the alteration of the female genitalia. Immediate health consequences include bleeding, infection and death. Longer-term damage and scarring can lead to incontinence, sexual dysfunction and difficulties in childbirth.

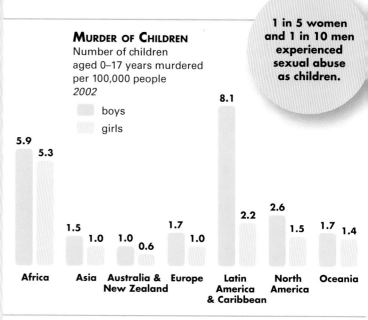

MURDER OF CHILDREN
Number of children aged 0–17 years murdered per 100,000 people
2002

boys
girls

Africa 5.9 / 5.3
Asia 1.5 / 1.0
Australia & New Zealand 1.0 / 0.6
Europe 1.7 / 1.0
Latin America & Caribbean 8.1 / 2.2
North America 2.6 / 1.5
Oceania 1.7 / 1.4

1 in 5 women and 1 in 10 men experienced sexual abuse as children.

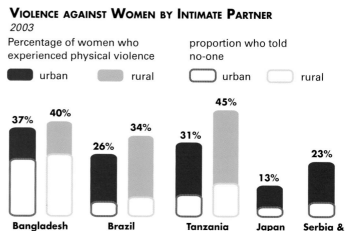

VIOLENCE AGAINST WOMEN BY INTIMATE PARTNER
2003

Percentage of women who experienced physical violence
■ urban   ▬ rural

proportion who told no-one
▭ urban   ▭ rural

Bangladesh 37% / 40%
Brazil 26% / 34%
Tanzania 31% / 45%
Japan 13%
Serbia & Montenegro 23%

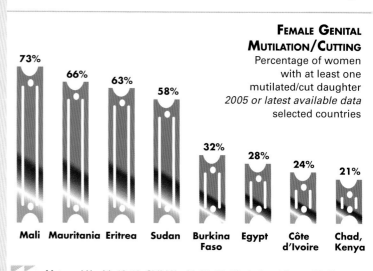

FEMALE GENITAL MUTILATION/CUTTING
Percentage of women with at least one mutilated/cut daughter
2005 or latest available data
selected countries

Mali 73%
Mauritania 66%
Eritrea 63%
Sudan 58%
Burkina Faso 32%
Egypt 28%
Côte d'Ivoire 24%
Chad, Kenya 21%

Maternal Health 18–19; Child Health 20–21; Alcohol and Drugs 40–41

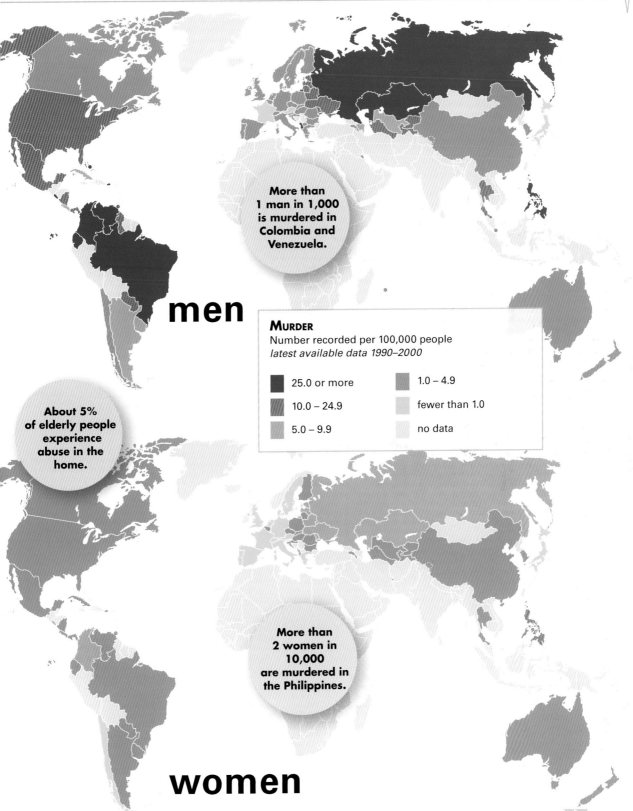

men

More than
1 man in 1,000
is murdered in
Colombia and
Venezuela.

MURDER
Number recorded per 100,000 people
latest available data 1990–2000

- 25.0 or more
- 10.0 – 24.9
- 5.0 – 9.9
- 1.0 – 4.9
- fewer than 1.0
- no data

About 5%
of elderly people
experience
abuse in the
home.

More than
2 women in
10,000
are murdered in
the Philippines.

women

Deaths from injuries accounted for 9 percent of deaths globally in 2000 and are increasing dramatically.

Unintentional injuries (from road traffic crashes, fires, poisoning, drowning, falls and other causes), and intentional injuries (from violence and abuse), kill more than 5 million people each year. Millions more are injured, some permanently disabled. As well as causing enormous suffering, this is a major drain on rehabilitation services and on healthcare resources in general.

The rate of injury varies across age groups. Eight of the 15 leading causes of death in people aged between 15 and 29 are injury related. In every country, injury and violence most adversely affect the poorest people – those whose conditions of living, working and travel are least safe, and whose access to prevention efforts and to care and rehabilitation is usually less than that of wealthier people.

Over 1 million people die, and up to 50 million are injured, in road-traffic crashes each year. These numbers are expected to rise by more than 60 percent by 2020 if current trends continue.

In the past, most injuries were regarded as the result of an "accident" – random and unavoidable – but now most are recognized as preventable. For example, interventions can reduce a number of the main causes of road crashes, including speed and alcohol limits, seat belts, helmets and visibility at night.

DEATHS FROM INJURY
Rate per 100,000 people
2000

men

women

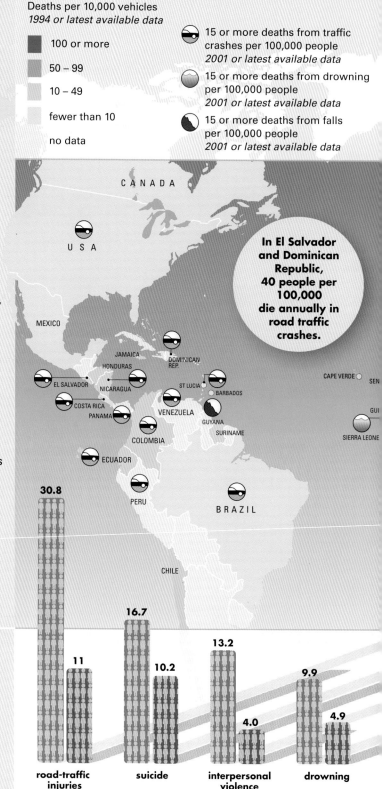

FATAL ROAD CRASHES
Deaths per 10,000 vehicles
1994 or latest available data

- 100 or more
- 50 – 99
- 10 – 49
- fewer than 10
- no data

15 or more deaths from traffic crashes per 100,000 people
2001 or latest available data

15 or more deaths from drowning per 100,000 people
2001 or latest available data

15 or more deaths from falls per 100,000 people
2001 or latest available data

In El Salvador and Dominican Republic, 40 people per 100,000 die annually in road traffic crashes.

Deaths from injury chart (rate per 100,000):
- road-traffic injuries: 30.8 / 11
- suicide: 16.7 / 10.2
- interpersonal violence: 13.2 / 4.0
- drowning: 9.9 / 4.9

Housing Conditions 32-33; Working Conditions 34-35; Alcohol and drugs 40-4
Violence and Abuse 52–53

VACCINE-PREVENTABLE DISEASES

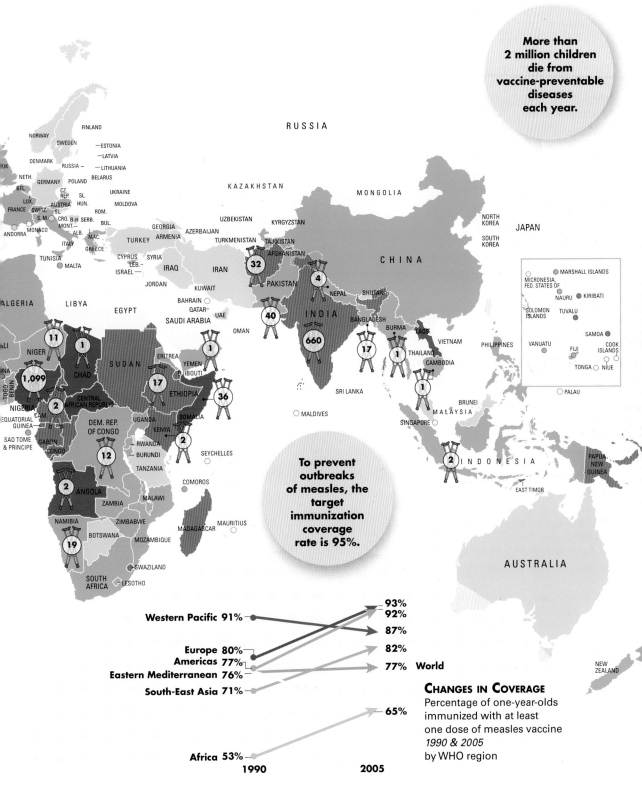

More than
2 million children
die from
vaccine-preventable
diseases
each year.

NORWAY
FINLAND
SWEDEN
DENMARK
ESTONIA
LATVIA
RUSSIA
LITHUANIA
BELARUS
NETH.
GERMANY POLAND
BEL
CZ. SL.
REP.
LUX.
AUSTRIA HUN.
FRANCE SWITZ. SL.
S. M. CRO. B-H SERB.
MONT.
ANDORRA MONACO ALB.
ITALY MAC.
GREECE

RUSSIA

KAZAKHSTAN

MONGOLIA

NORTH
KOREA

JAPAN

SOUTH
KOREA

UKRAINE
MOLDOVA
ROM.
BUL.
GEORGIA
ARMENIA AZERBAIJAN
TURKEY
UZBEKISTAN
KYRGYZSTAN
TURKMENISTAN
TAJIKISTAN
32
AFGHANISTAN
4
NEPAL BHUTAN
CHINA

TUNISIA
MALTA
CYPRUS SYRIA
LEB.
ISRAEL
IRAQ
IRAN
JORDAN
KUWAIT
BAHRAIN
QATAR
UAE
SAUDI ARABIA
OMAN
PAKISTAN
40
INDIA
660
BANGLADESH
BURMA
17
LAOS
1
THAILAND
VIETNAM
CAMBODIA
1

ALGERIA
LIBYA
EGYPT

MARSHALL ISLANDS
MICRONESIA,
FED. STATES OF
NAURU KIRIBATI
SOLOMON
ISLANDS
TUVALU
SAMOA
PHILIPPINES
VANUATU
FIJI
COOK
ISLANDS
TONGA NIUE
PALAU

11
NIGER
1
CHAD
SUDAN
ERITREA
1
YEMEN
DJIBOUTI
17
ETHIOPIA
36
1,099
NIGERIA
CAM.
2
CENTRAL
AFRICAN REPUBLIC
SOMALIA
EQUATORIAL
GUINEA
SAO TOME
& PRINCIPE
GABON
CONGO
DEM. REP.
OF CONGO
UGANDA
KENYA
2
RWANDA
BURUNDI
12
TANZANIA
SEYCHELLES

SRI LANKA
MALDIVES
BRUNEI
MALAYSIA
SINGAPORE

To prevent
outbreaks
of measles, the
target
immunization
coverage
rate is 95%.

2 INDONESIA
EAST TIMOR
PAPUA
NEW
GUINEA

2 ANGOLA
ZAMBIA
MALAWI
COMOROS
MADAGASCAR
MAURITIUS
NAMIBIA
ZIMBABWE
BOTSWANA
MOZAMBIQUE
19
SWAZILAND
SOUTH
AFRICA
LESOTHO

AUSTRALIA

CHANGES IN COVERAGE

Western Pacific 91%
93%
92%
87%

Europe 80%
Americas 77%
Eastern Mediterranean 76%
82%
77% World

South-East Asia 71%

65%

Percentage of one-year-olds
immunized with at least
one dose of measles vaccine
1990 & 2005
by WHO region

NEW
ZEALAND

Africa 53%
1990
2005

Prevalence of sexually transmitted infections (STIs) is increasing in most countries.

Many organisms can be transmitted sexually. Common curable STIs include syphilis, gonorrhoea, chlamydia and the parasite trichomoniasis. Viral STIs include HIV, herpes, human papilloma virus (HPV) and hepatitis B. Some of these infections may not have symptoms, making detection, diagnosis, management, control and surveillance very difficult. The risk of acquiring STIs is highest in the young and the poor in urban areas.

The prevention and control of STIs reduces related morbidity, long-term disability and death. For women, it prevents serious complications, including ectopic pregnancy and infertility. It also prevents miscarriages, stillbirths, pre-term deliveries, low birth-weight and congenital infections in newborns that can lead to death or complications such as blindness. Prevention of HPV protects against cervical cancer, the second commonest cause of cancer death in women worldwide.

STIs increase the risk of HIV transmission. Condoms are the only contraceptive method proven to reduce the risk of STIs, including HIV. Promotion of safer sexual behaviour, and encouragement to seek treatment at an early stage of infection is a vital part of STI prevention and care. Other preventive strategies include sexual abstinence, the delaying of first sexual experiences and a reduction in the number of sexual partners.

Integrated sexual and reproductive health services, and comprehensive case management through multidisciplinary control are needed to ensure correct diagnosis and treatment, education on prevention of transmission, and on tracing, treating and counselling sexual partners. Because surveillance of STIs is inadequate in many places, prevalence data are limited. Research continues for ways to improve diagnosis and treatment, develop preventive vaccines and modify sexual behaviour.

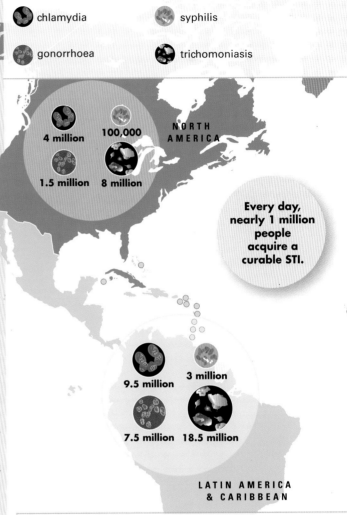

CURABLE STIs
Estimated number of new cases of selected STIs
1999
by WHO sub-region

- chlamydia
- gonorrhoea
- syphilis
- trichomoniasis

4 million
100,000
NORTH AMERICA
1.5 million
8 million

Every day, nearly 1 million people acquire a curable STI.

9.5 million
3 million
7.5 million
18.5 million

LATIN AMERICA & CARIBBEAN

CONDOM USE
Percentage of males aged 15–24 years using condom for higher-risk sex
2005 or latest available data
selected countries

Madagascar	Chad	Haiti	Mozambique	Bolivia	Kenya, Mali
12%	25%	30%	33%	37%	47%

Maternal Health 18–19; Child Health 20–21; Education 26–27

SEXUALLY TRANSMITTED INFECTIONS

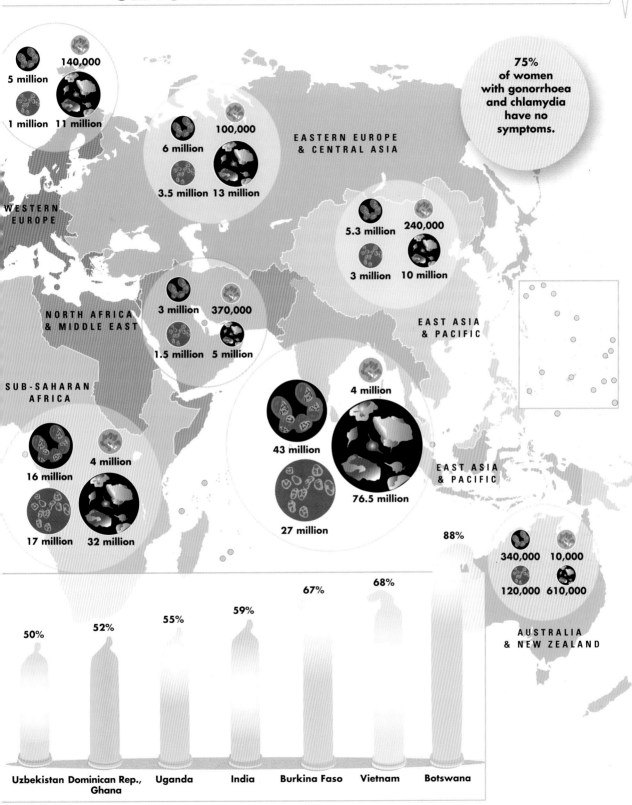

140,000

5 million

1 million   11 million

75%
of women
with gonorrhoea
and chlamydia
have no
symptoms.

EASTERN EUROPE
& CENTRAL ASIA

100,000

6 million

3.5 million   13 million

WESTERN
EUROPE

5.3 million   **240,000**

3 million   10 million

NORTH AFRICA
& MIDDLE EAST

3 million   **370,000**

1.5 million   5 million

EAST ASIA
& PACIFIC

SUB-SAHARAN
AFRICA

4 million

16 million

4 million

17 million   32 million

43 million

76.5 million

27 million

EAST ASIA
& PACIFIC

88%

340,000   **10,000**

120,000   610,000

AUSTRALIA
& NEW ZEALAND

67%   68%

59%

55%

52%

50%

Uzbekistan   Dominican Rep.,   Uganda   India   Burkina Faso   Vietnam   Botswana
Ghana

HIV deaths and new infections continue to increase.

HIV/AIDS is one of the greatest development and security issues facing the world today. Since it was first recognized in 1981, AIDS has killed more than 25 million people, and more than 65 million people have been infected with HIV. Two-thirds of all people living with HIV are in Sub-Saharan Africa, and most do not know that they have the infection. Growing epidemics are also underway in China, India and Eastern Europe.

Since the late 1990s, anti-retroviral (ARV) therapy has transformed the lives of people with HIV infection who have access to it. AIDS-related deaths have plummeted in rich countries. While enormous efforts are being made to expand access to these treatments in resource-poor countries, profound inequalities in access remain. In Africa, fewer women than men receive ARV.

Voluntary counselling and testing is essential to controlling the disease. Around 1,500 infants become infected with HIV each day, but in 2005 only 9 percent of pregnant women in low- and middle-income countries were offered services to prevent transmission to their newborns.

Fifteen million children under the age of 18 have lost one or both parents to AIDS, leaving them particularly vulnerable and less likely to attend school. Some of them have been born with HIV infection. Limited access to healthcare, education and social support worsens the effects of their poverty, and in many settings they are at high risk of sexual exploitation and of further exposure to HIV.

Research continues into new preventive technologies, including vaccines and microbicides. Efforts at prevention and treatment must be both scaled up and intensified to stop millions of new infections occurring.

PREVALENCE OF HIV INFECTION

Percentage of persons aged 15–49 infected with HIV
end 2005 estimates

- 20.0% and over
- 10.0% – 19.9%
- 1.0% – 9.9%
- fewer than 1%
- no data

Number of AIDS orphans
- 1 million or more
- 100,000 – 999,999

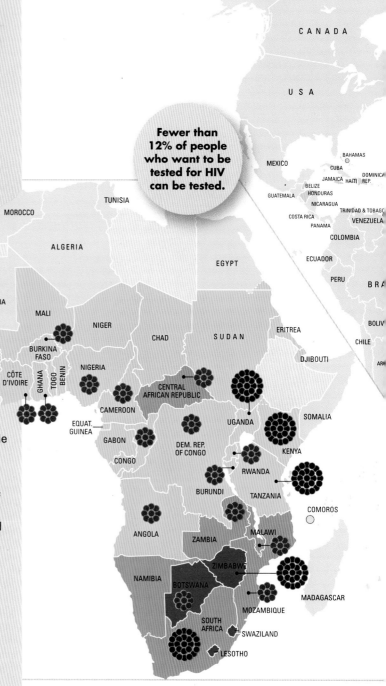

Fewer than 12% of people who want to be tested for HIV can be tested.

Life Expectancy 16–17; Sexually Transmitted Diseases 62–63

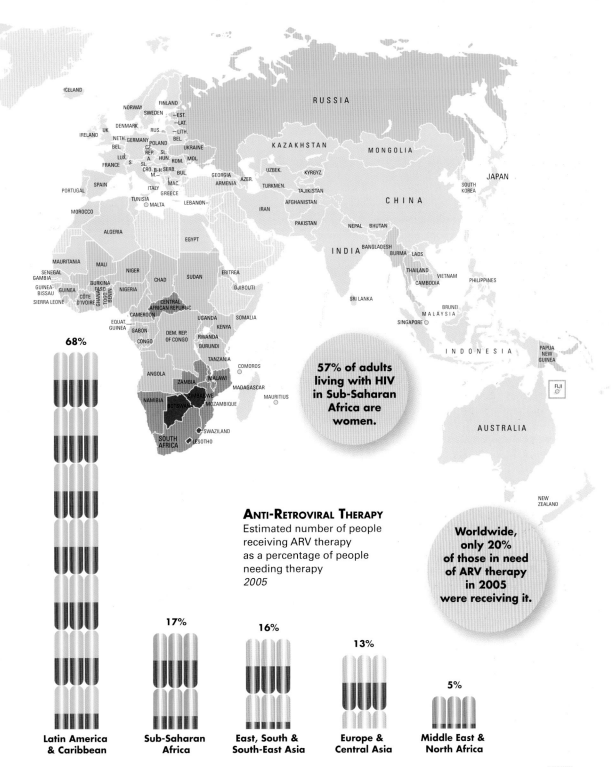

HIV/AIDS

57% of adults living with HIV in Sub-Saharan Africa are women.

Worldwide, only 20% of those in need of ARV therapy in 2005 were receiving it.

ANTI-RETROVIRAL THERAPY

Estimated number of people receiving ARV therapy as a percentage of people needing therapy
2005

68%
Latin America & Caribbean

17%
Sub-Saharan Africa

16%
East, South & South-East Asia

13%
Europe & Central Asia

5%
Middle East & North Africa

Despite being preventable and curable, TB continues to be a leading global cause of death and disability.

One person in three is estimated to be infected with TB. In most cases the disease is latent, but in 5 to 10 percent the disease will become active at some point, and, if untreated, infectious. A person with active TB typically infects 15 people a year, who breathe in bacteria-carrying droplets exhaled or coughed by the sufferer.

Even though new TB cases and TB deaths are declining slightly worldwide, they are increasing in Africa and South-East Asia. TB can be difficult to diagnose and treat. The introduction of DOTS (directly observed treatment) in the mid-1990s has led to high cure rates and successful prevention of new infections, but it requires strong health systems, especially in primary care. TB is also a major cause of death among people with HIV/AIDS.

TB is becoming more dangerous because of the emergence of multi-drug-resistant TB (MDR-TB), which does not respond to the standard drug treatments, and is being increasingly reported around the world. Extensively drug-resistant TB (XDR-TB) is a newly identified global threat in which patients (many of whom are also living with HIV) are virtually untreatable using currently available drugs. Strengthening of health systems for TB and HIV control, including better prevention, diagnosis, treatment, and surveillance are essential to limit the spread of drug-resistant infections.

New vaccines for prevention, improved diagnostic tests for identification and new drugs for treatment are urgently needed.

TB PREVALENCE
Cases per 100,000 people
2005

- 500 or more
- 300 – 499
- 100 – 299
- 50 – 99
- fewer than 50
- no data

TB deaths among HIV-positive people exceed 40 per 100,000 people
2004–05

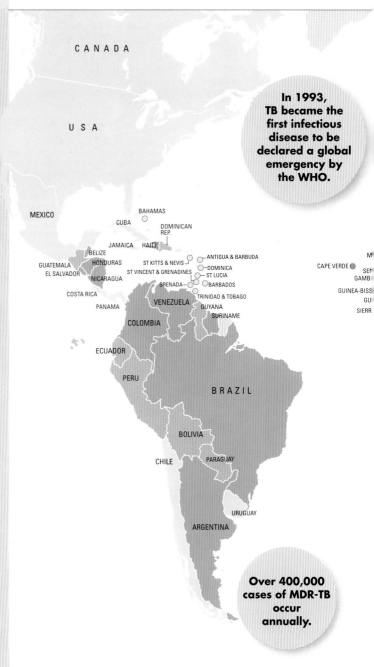

In 1993, TB became the first infectious disease to be declared a global emergency by the WHO.

Over 400,000 cases of MDR-TB occur annually.

Life Expectancy 16-17; Healthcare 36–37; HIV/AIDS 64–65

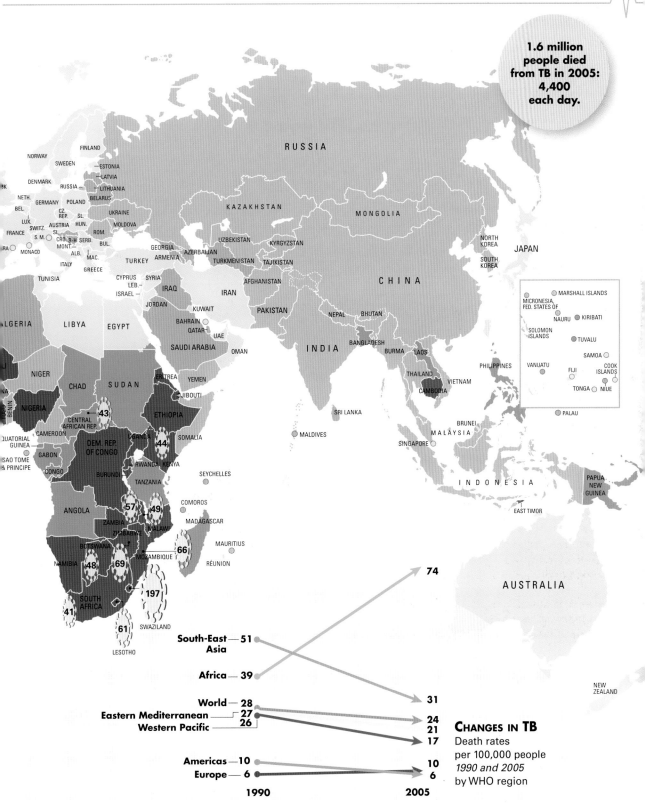

1.6 million people died from TB in 2005: 4,400 each day.

NORWAY
SWEDEN
FINLAND
DENMARK
RUSSIA
NETH.
GERMANY POLAND
BEL.
CZ.
LUX. REP.
SWITZ. AUSTRIA HUN.
FRANCE S.M.
MONACO CRO. B-H SERB.
MONT.
ITALY ALB. MAC.
GREECE
TUNISIA
ESTONIA
LATVIA
LITHUANIA
BELARUS
UKRAINE
SL. MOLDOVA
ROM.
BUL.
GEORGIA
ARMENIA AZERBAIJAN
CYPRUS SYRIA
LEB.
ISRAEL IRAQ
JORDAN
BAHRAIN
QATAR
UAE
SAUDI ARABIA
OMAN
YEMEN

RUSSIA

KAZAKHSTAN

MONGOLIA

UZBEKISTAN KYRGYZSTAN
TURKMENISTAN TAJIKISTAN

AFGHANISTAN

TURKEY

IRAN

KUWAIT

PAKISTAN

NEPAL BHUTAN

INDIA

BANGLADESH

BURMA

SRI LANKA

MALDIVES

NORTH KOREA

SOUTH KOREA

JAPAN

CHINA

LAOS
THAILAND
VIETNAM
CAMBODIA

PHILIPPINES

BRUNEI
MALAYSIA

SINGAPORE

INDONESIA

EAST TIMOR

MARSHALL ISLANDS
MICRONESIA,
FED. STATES OF
NAURU KIRIBATI
SOLOMON ISLANDS
TUVALU
SAMOA
VANUATU
FIJI
TONGA NIUE
COOK ISLANDS
PALAU

LGERIA LIBYA EGYPT
NIGER CHAD SUDAN
ERITREA
DJIBOUTI
ETHIOPIA
SOMALIA
NIGERIA
BENIN
CENTRAL
AFRICAN REP.
CAMEROON
QUATORIAL GUINEA
SAO TOME & PRINCIPE
GABON CONGO
UGANDA
DEM. REP. OF CONGO
RWANDA KENYA
BURUNDI
TANZANIA
SEYCHELLES
COMOROS
ANGOLA
ZAMBIA
ZIMBABWE
MALAWI
BOTSWANA
MADAGASCAR
MAURITIUS
RÉUNION
NAMIBIA
MOZAMBIQUE
SOUTH AFRICA
SWAZILAND
LESOTHO

43
44
57 **49**
66
48 **69**
197
41
61

PAPUA NEW GUINEA

AUSTRALIA

NEW ZEALAND

74

31

24
21
17

10
6

South-East — 51
Asia

Africa — 39

World — 28
Eastern Mediterranean — 27
Western Pacific — 26

Americas — 10
Europe — 6

1990

2005

CHANGES IN TB
Death rates
per 100,000 people
1990 and 2005
by WHO region

Malaria is preventable and curable, but continues to be a major obstacle to social and economic development.

There are an estimated 500 million cases of malaria each year, resulting in over 1 million deaths, the majority of them in Sub-Saharan Africa. Malaria is caused by *Plasmodium* parasites, which are transmitted from person to person by the bites of infected mosquitoes (the vector). Around 40 percent of people live in areas where malaria is a risk.

Malaria has an enormous impact on households and healthcare systems in affected regions. It is estimated to cost Africa over US$12 billion a year in lost GDP, even though it could be controlled for a fraction of that sum.

The poor are especially affected as they have least access to effective services, information, and protective measures. Children, pregnant women and migrating populations are most vulnerable. Malaria in pregnancy causes death, anaemia, miscarriage, stillbirth, and low birth-weight.

An effective vaccine would be a major contribution to malaria prevention and control, but although research continues, this is not expected to be available for some years. Drug resistance is widespread, mainly due to past use of inappropriate drugs. New drugs are being developed, but many are too expensive for individuals or governments in poorer countries. Cost-effective interventions include rapid diagnosis and prompt treatment, the use of insecticide-treated nets (ITNs), and the control of the mosquito by use of indoor sprays.

If a sufficient proportion of a community is protected, the *Plasmodium* parasite's route from insect to person to insect to the next person is interrupted, and death rates decline.

The extent of malaria episodes and deaths is uncertain because of inadequate health reporting systems, and the fact that the co-incidence of malaria with other diseases can make it difficult to diagnose.

CHILD DEATHS FROM MALARIA
Percentage of deaths in under-fives caused by malaria
2000

- 20.0% or more
- 10.0 – 19.9%
- 1.0% – 9.9%
- fewer than 1.0%
- none
- no data

50% or more of under-fives with fever receiving anti-malarial treatment *2004 or latest available data*

33% or more of under-fives sleeping under an insecticide treated net *2004 or latest available data*

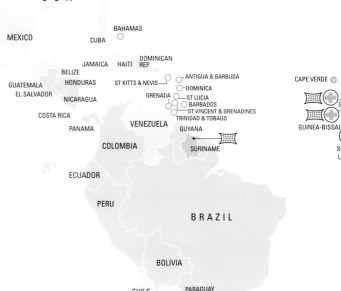

A child dies of malaria every 30 seconds.

Maternal Health 18–19; Child Health 20–21; Housing 32–33; Healthcare 36–37

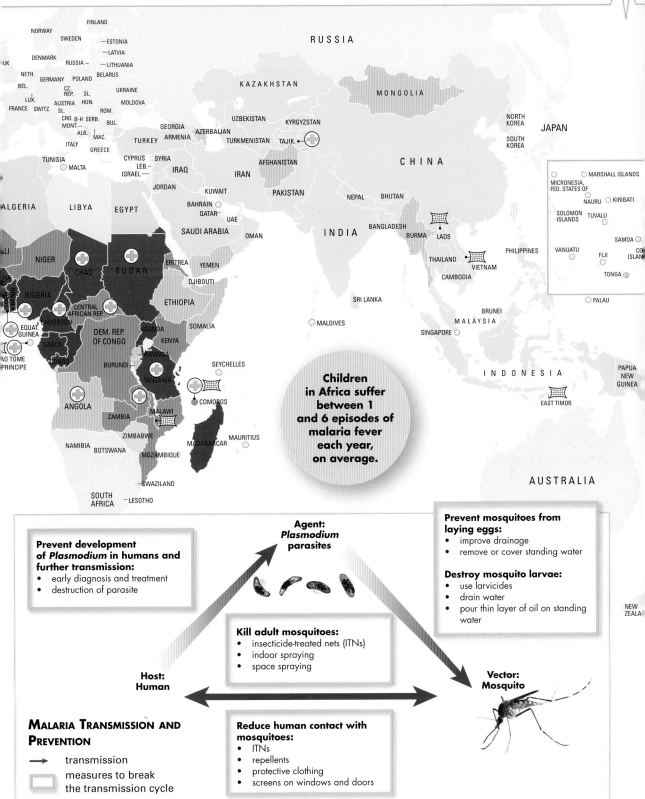

FINLAND
NORWAY
SWEDEN — ESTONIA
— LATVIA
RUSSIA — — LITHUANIA
DENMARK BELARUS
UK
NETH. GERMANY POLAND
BEL. CZ. SL. UKRAINE
LUX. REP. HUN.
AUSTRIA MOLDOVA
FRANCE SWITZ. CRO. B-H SERB. ROM.
MONT.— BUL.
ALB. MAC.
ITALY GREECE
TUNISIA CYPRUS SYRIA
MALTA LEB.– IRAQ
ISRAEL — JORDAN

RUSSIA

KAZAKHSTAN

MONGOLIA

NORTH
KOREA
JAPAN
SOUTH
KOREA

GEORGIA
AZERBAIJAN
TURKEY ARMENIA
TURKMENISTAN TAJIK.

UZBEKISTAN KYRGYZSTAN

C H I N A

AFGHANISTAN

KUWAIT
BAHRAIN
QATAR
UAE
SAUDI ARABIA
OMAN

IRAN
PAKISTAN

NEPAL BHUTAN
BANGLADESH
I N D I A BURMA LAOS
THAILAND
VIETNAM
CAMBODIA

MICRONESIA,
FED. STATES OF

MARSHALL ISLANDS

NAURU KIRIBATI
SOLOMON TUVALU
ISLANDS
SAMOA CO
VANUATU ISLAN
FIJI
TONGA

ALGERIA LIBYA EGYPT

MALI
NIGER CHAD SUDAN ERITREA YEMEN
NIGERIA DJIBOUTI
CENTRAL ETHIOPIA
CAMEROON AFRICAN REP
EQUAT. UGANDA SOMALIA
GUINEA DEM. REP. KENYA
GABON OF CONGO
AO TOME CONGO RWANDA
PRINCIPE BURUNDI TANZANIA
ANGOLA
ZAMBIA MALAWI
ZIMBABWE
NAMIBIA MOZAMBIQUE
BOTSWANA
SWAZILAND
SOUTH — LESOTHO
AFRICA

SRI LANKA

MALDIVES

SEYCHELLES

COMOROS

MADAGASCAR MAURITIUS

PALAU

BRUNEI
M A L A Y S I A
SINGAPORE

I N D O N E S I A

EAST TIMOR

PHILIPPINES

PAPUA
NEW
GUINEA

Children in Africa suffer between 1 and 6 episodes of malaria fever each year, on average.

A U S T R A L I A

NEW
ZEALA

Prevent development of *Plasmodium* in humans and further transmission:
- early diagnosis and treatment
- destruction of parasite

Agent:
***Plasmodium* parasites**

Prevent mosquitoes from laying eggs:
- improve drainage
- remove or cover standing water

Destroy mosquito larvae:
- use larvicides
- drain water
- pour thin layer of oil on standing water

Kill adult mosquitoes:
- insecticide-treated nets (ITNs)
- indoor spraying
- space spraying

Host:
Human

Vector:
Mosquito

MALARIA TRANSMISSION AND PREVENTION

→ transmission

measures to break the transmission cycle

Reduce human contact with mosquitoes:
- ITNs
- repellents
- protective clothing
- screens on windows and doors

NEW
ZEALA

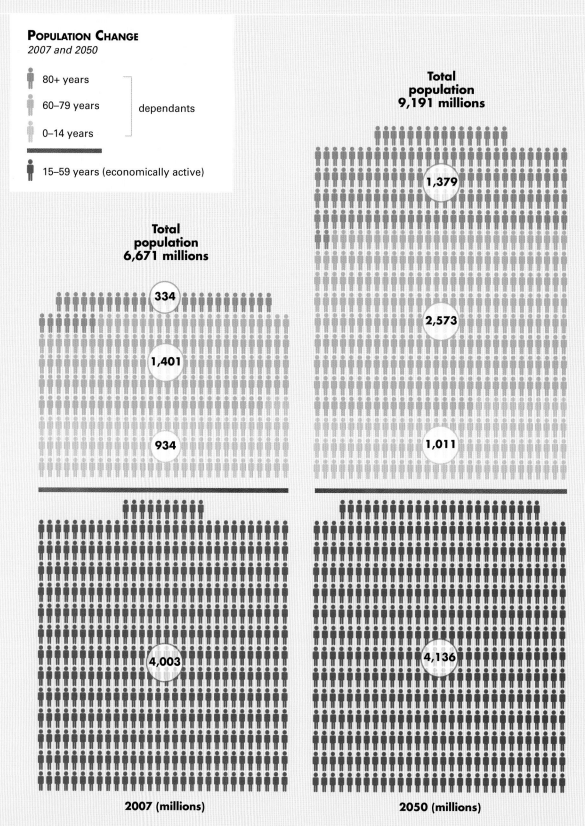

POPULATION CHANGE
2007 and 2050

- 80+ years
- 60–79 years } dependants
- 0–14 years

- 15–59 years (economically active)

Total population 9,191 millions

1,379

2,573

1,011

Total population 6,671 millions

334

1,401

934

4,003

4,136

2007 (millions)

2050 (millions)

PART 4

PUBLIC HEALTH CHALLENGES

As the world's population grows, and as people live longer, we need to prepare for enormous changes in the health issues that will have to be addressed. A growing and ageing population will require new policies and programmes to deal with the expected changes to the prevalence and pattern of disease and health problems. More skilled workers will be needed in health systems that are currently under-resourced to deal with these emerging issues.

Maternal mortality, malnutrition and communicable diseases will continue to be major problems for people living in low-income countries, while non-communicable diseases and injuries will become increasing problems in all parts of the world. Emerging infectious diseases, antimicrobial resistance and the threat of a pandemic of influenza or another infection are concerns everywhere, and are likely to be compounded by an increasingly mobile global population. Rapid urbanization and the impact of climate change, and the consequences of both on people's health, need to be addressed at international, national and local levels.

As people migrate from rural to urban settings they are exposed to new health risks.

The urban share of the population is growing faster than ever before, especially in Africa and Asia. In 1950, New York was the only megacity – a metropolitan area with a population greater than 10 million people – but most of the megacities that have grown since then have been in low- or middle-income countries. It is predicted that, by 2030, 80 percent of urban dwellers will live in towns and cities in developing countries. Many will be living in slums – part of the trend towards the urbanization of poverty.

Inadequate shelter is a central feature of urban poverty. Adequate housing provides security and safety, a basis for social networks and a means of access to basic services. The urban poor are at risk from low-quality, poorly ventilated, overcrowded living and working conditions, from indoor and outdoor air pollution, lack of safe drinking water, sanitation and basic services, and from limited access to education and health services.

Inadequate nutrition leaves people more at risk from infectious diseases, including waterborne diseases and opportunistic infections associated with HIV infection, which are more common in slum areas. Women and children are especially vulnerable. Cities contribute to environmental damage through pollution, resource degradation and waste generation, all of which facilitate the spread of disease.

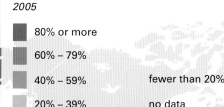

URBAN DWELLERS
As percentage of total population
2005

- 80% or more
- 60% – 79%
- 40% – 59%
- 20% – 39%
- fewer than 20%
- no data

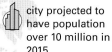

MEGACITIES

city with population over 10 million in 2005

city projected to have population over 10 million in 2015

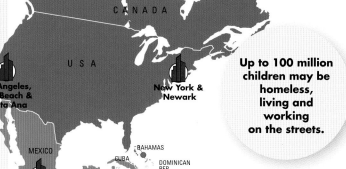

Up to 100 million children may be homeless, living and working on the streets.

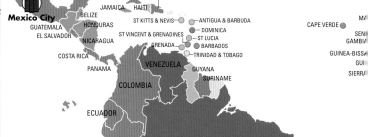

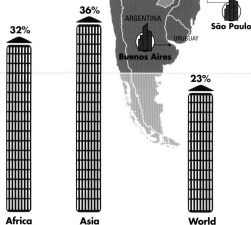

32%
36%
23%

URBANIZATION
Projected percentage increase in urban dwellers as share of population
2005–30

4%
Oceania

7%
North America

8%
Europe

9%
Latin America & Caribbean

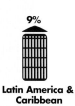
Africa

Asia

World

Housing Conditions 32–33; Working Conditions 34–35; Respiratory Diseases 5

URBANIZATION

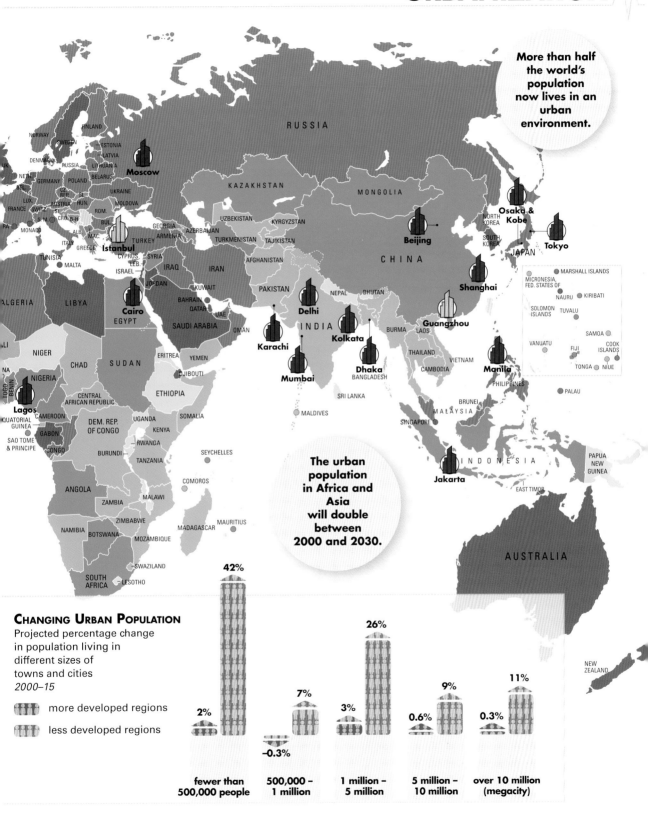

More than half the world's population now lives in an urban environment.

RUSSIA

NORWAY
SWEDEN
FINLAND
DENMARK
ESTONIA
LATVIA
LITHUANIA
RUSSIA
BELARUS
POLAND
GERMANY
NETH.
BEL.
LUX.
CZ.
AUSTRIA
HUN.
FRANCE
SWITZ.
S.M.
CRO.
B-H
MONACO
ITALY
ALB.
MAC.
GREECE
TUNISIA
MALTA

Moscow

KAZAKHSTAN
UZBEKISTAN
KYRGYZSTAN
TURKMENISTAN
TAJIKISTAN

MONGOLIA

NORTH KOREA
SOUTH KOREA
JAPAN

Osaka & Kobe

Tokyo

GEORGIA
ARMENIA
AZERBAIJAN
AFGHANISTAN

Istanbul
TURKEY
CYPRUS
LEB.
SYRIA
IRAQ
IRAN
JORDAN
ISRAEL
KUWAIT
BAHRAIN
QATAR
UAE
OMAN

Cairo
EGYPT
SAUDI ARABIA

PAKISTAN
NEPAL
BHUTAN

CHINA

Beijing

Shanghai

MARSHALL ISLANDS
MICRONESIA, FED. STATES OF
NAURU
KIRIBATI
SOLOMON ISLANDS
TUVALU
SAMOA
VANUATU
FIJI
COOK ISLANDS
TONGA
NIUE
PALAU

ALGERIA
LIBYA

NIGER
CHAD
SUDAN
ERITREA
YEMEN
DJIBOUTI

Delhi

Karachi
INDIA

Kolkata

BURMA
LAOS

Guangzhou

THAILAND
VIETNAM
CAMBODIA

Mumbai

Dhaka
BANGLADESH

SRI LANKA

Manila
PHILIPPINES

NIGERIA
BENIN
TOGO

Lagos
EQUATORIAL GUINEA
CAMEROON
CENTRAL AFRICAN REPUBLIC
ETHIOPIA
SOMALIA
UGANDA
KENYA

DEM. REP. OF CONGO
GABON
CONGO
SAO TOME & PRINCIPE
RWANDA
BURUNDI
TANZANIA

MALDIVES

BRUNEI
MALAYSIA
SINGAPORE

SEYCHELLES

ANGOLA
ZAMBIA
MALAWI
COMOROS

NAMIBIA
ZIMBABWE
BOTSWANA
MOZAMBIQUE
MADAGASCAR
MAURITIUS

The urban population in Africa and Asia will double between 2000 and 2030.

INDONESIA

Jakarta

EAST TIMOR

PAPUA NEW GUINEA

AUSTRALIA

SWAZILAND
SOUTH AFRICA
LESOTHO

NEW ZEALAND

CHANGING URBAN POPULATION
Projected percentage change in population living in different sizes of towns and cities
2000–15

more developed regions

less developed regions

42%

26%

2%

7%

3%

0.6%

9%

0.3%

11%

-0.3%

fewer than 500,000 people

500,000 – 1 million

1 million – 5 million

5 million – 10 million

over 10 million (megacity)

Climate change is likely to have an adverse effect on health, especially among the poorest, most vulnerable populations.

The 2007 report of the Intergovernmental Panel on Climate Change (IPCC) assessed the likelihood of human activities being the cause of climate change as more than 90 percent. The emission of greenhouse gases from the burning of fossil fuels has led to a rise in global temperatures, which is predicted to result in increased rainfall in high-latitude countries, and increased frequency and intensity of droughts in the tropics.

Some favourable effects on health are predicted, such as a reduction in cold-related deaths in temperate climates, and an increase in food production in some high-latitude regions. Serious negative effects are also expected as a result of unsafe drinking water, inadequate food, lack of secure shelter, and changes in disease patterns.

The greatest adverse impact will undoubtedly be felt in low-income countries, which have produced the lowest greenhouse emissions, and where the capacity to adapt and to mitigate the effect of climate change is weakest.

The risks associated with climate change need to be included in health surveillance systems, and in emergency planning and preparedness. Reducing the risks by reducing greenhouse gas emissions is essential for health.

HEALTH IMPACT OF CLIMATE

Annual number of DALYs per million people from malnutrition, diarrhoea, flooding, and malaria caused by climate-related conditions
2000 by WHO region

- more than 3,000
- 1,500 – 3,000
- 100 – 199
- under 10
- no data

total annual DALYs

DALYs or disability adjusted life years are the number of years of potential life lost due to premature mortality, plus years of productive life lost due to disability.

The global average surface temperature increased by 0.6°C during the 20th century.

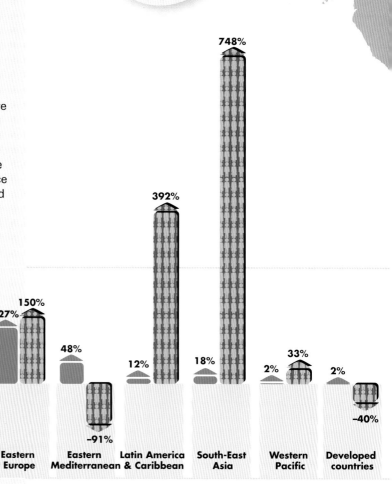

92,000

LATIN AMERICA AND CARIBBEAN

EXTREME WEATHER EVENTS

Percentage change in number of events and in number of people killed
1980s – 1990s

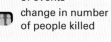

change in number of events

change in number of people killed

Region	change in events	change in people killed
Africa	2%	–98%
Eastern Europe	127%	150%
Eastern Mediterranean	48%	–91%
Latin America & Caribbean	12%	392%
South-East Asia	18%	748%
Western Pacific	2%	33%
Developed countries	2%	–40%

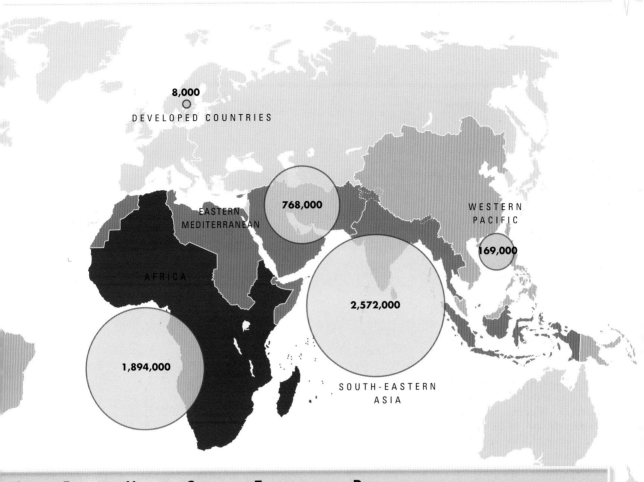

8,000
DEVELOPED COUNTRIES

768,000
EASTERN
MEDITERRANEAN

WESTERN
PACIFIC

169,000

AFRICA

2,572,000

1,894,000

SOUTH-EASTERN
ASIA

ADVERSE EFFECTS ON HEALTH OF CHANGES IN TEMPERATURE AND RAINFALL

Environmental change	Health effects
Increase in temperature	Vector-borne diseases, such as malaria and dengue, spreading to previously unaffected areas, and changing their seasonal pattern.
Increased frequency of heatwaves and droughts	Increase in deaths and morbidity related to heat and dehydration, particularly among most vulnerable. Increase in malnutrition from food shortages. Increase in pollen and dust. Adverse health effects of population displacement.
Increased frequency of storms and floods	Increase in deaths from drowning. Increase in injuries. Increase in morbidity from diarrhoeal and waterborne diseases, sewage contamination and salinity of soil. Adverse health effects of population displacement.
Increase in air pollution	Increase in cardio-respiratory disease from higher ground-level ozone, pollens, dust.
Rise in sea-level	Flooding. Increase in disease as a result of contamination of water supplies. Adverse health effects of population displacement.

War accounts for more death and disability than many major diseases.

The majority of the dead and injured are usually civilians, although calculating deaths is difficult when vital registrations systems are disrupted or limited. Long-term mental health problems affect both military and civilians. Landmines can continue to kill and maim for years after conflict has ended. Rape is used as a weapon of war.

Armed conflict and war account for most of the world's refugees, asylum seekers and internally displaced people, many of whom are living in crowded, unhygienic, and impoverished conditions, with inadequate shelter and sanitation. They are at increased risk of malnutrition, injuries and attacks, and of infectious diseases, including cholera and measles.

Where conflict occurs, the infrastructure to support health services may be damaged. Measures such as economic sanctions, and the deliberate destruction of healthcare facilities, food supplies, water treatment, sanitation, and transport and communication systems can all increase the risk of disease.

One of the indirect effects of war or civil unrest is the diversion of resources from healthcare and health-supporting social services towards expenditure on armaments and military forces. Being in a state of war can also lead to a population experiencing increased community and domestic violence, and environmental pollution and degradation.

Children in conflict situations are especially vulnerable to malnutrition, disease and injury. Some are forced to become child soldiers.

PEOPLE OF CONCERN TO THE UNHCR
Number of refugees, asylum seekers and internally displaced persons
2006

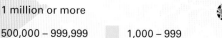

- 1 million or more
- 500,000 – 999,999
- 100,000 – 499,999
- 10,000 – 99,999
- 1,000 – 999
- fewer than 1,000
- no data

POLITICAL VIOLENCE

1,000 or more deaths from political violence *2006*

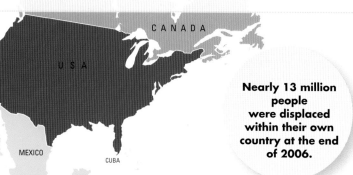

Nearly 13 million people were displaced within their own country at the end of 2006.

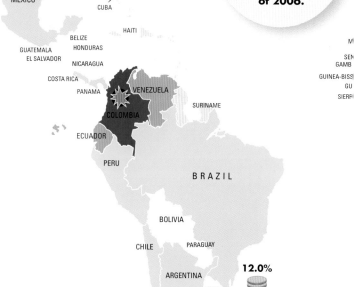

BATTLE-DEATHS
Regional distribution of deaths in battle of combatants and civilians *1990–2005*

Middle East 7%
Americas 5%
Europe 16%
Africa 49%
Asia 23%

Total: 1.2 million

12.0%
8.3%
2.7%
2.5%
Oman
Saudi Arabia

Violence and Abuse 52–53; Injury 54–55

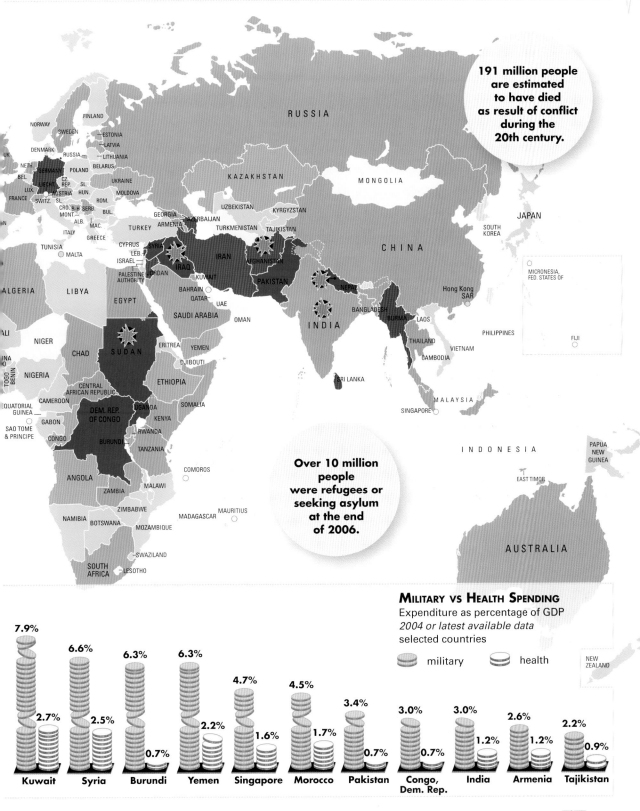

191 million people are estimated to have died as result of conflict during the 20th century.

Over 10 million people were refugees or seeking asylum at the end of 2006.

MILITARY VS HEALTH SPENDING
Expenditure as percentage of GDP
2004 or latest available data
selected countries

military   health

	Kuwait	Syria	Burundi	Yemen	Singapore	Morocco	Pakistan	Congo, Dem. Rep.	India	Armenia	Tajikistan
military	7.9%	6.6%	6.3%	6.3%	4.7%	4.5%	3.4%	3.0%	3.0%	2.6%	2.2%
health	2.7%	2.5%	0.7%	2.2%	1.6%	1.7%	0.7%	0.7%	1.2%	1.2%	0.9%

A severe influenza pandemic would result in a global crisis.

A pandemic is a severe outbreak of infectious disease that rapidly spreads to involve all parts of the world, with the potential to cause widespread human suffering and economic and social disruption.

Influenza outbreaks usually occur in the winter months in temperate regions, causing a seasonal increase in morbidity and mortality, particularly among the elderly, and people with decreased immunity. When a new strain of influenza virus appears to which the overall population has no immunity, a pandemic may result. With increasing international travel, a new virus could spread very rapidly.

In the pandemic of 1918–19, all age groups were affected, but there was particularly high mortality among healthy young adults. Further influenza pandemics occurred in 1957 (severe) and 1968 (moderate). As it is 50 years since the last severe pandemic, it is likely that the world's population would have little or no immunity to a new pandemic influenza strain, making a severe pandemic more likely. In 2003, the outbreak of the highly pathogenic avian influenza type H5N1 in birds went on to infect humans, causing severe disease with high death rates. There is real concern that if the virus were to mutate into a form more readily transmitted from human to human, it would cause a pandemic.

The outbreak of severe acute respiratory syndrome which began in 2002, caused by SARS coronavirus, has clearly demonstrated the need for a co-ordinated global response to a new, rapidly spreading infectious disease. Local transmission was demonstrated in a small number of countries; in the other places reporting the disease, the infection was shown to have travelled into the country from elsewhere.

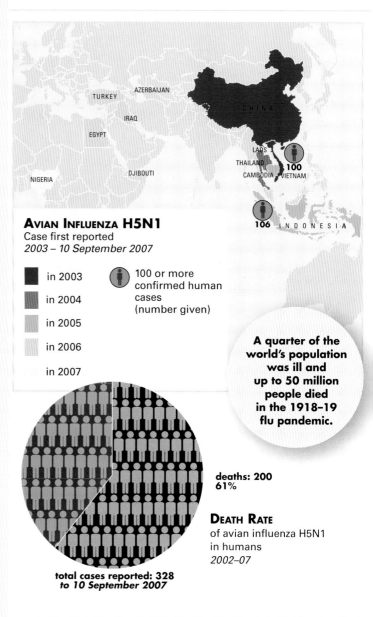

AVIAN INFLUENZA H5N1
Case first reported
2003 – 10 September 2007

- in 2003
- in 2004
- in 2005
- in 2006
- in 2007

100 or more confirmed human cases (number given)

A quarter of the world's population was ill and up to 50 million people died in the 1918–19 flu pandemic.

deaths: 200
61%

DEATH RATE
of avian influenza H5N1 in humans
2002–07

total cases reported: 328
to 10 September 2007

PHASES OF PANDEMIC ALERT

Phase 1	Phase 2
Low risk of human cases	Higher risk of human cases

INTER-PANDEMIC PHASE
New virus in animals, no human cases.

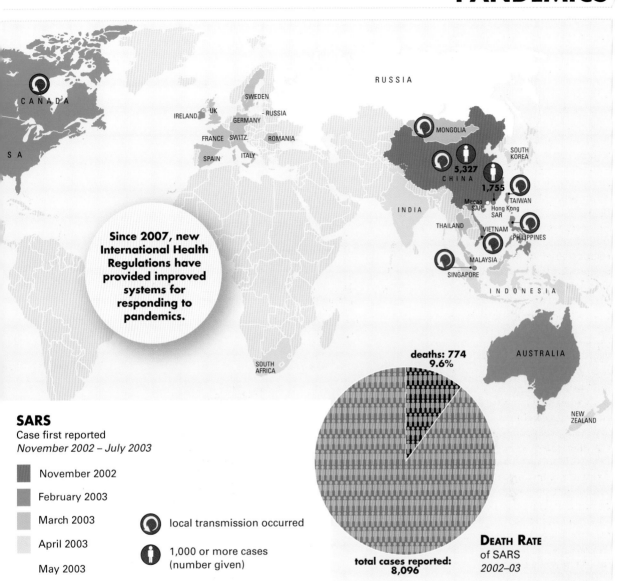

RUSSIA

SWEDEN
IRELAND — UK — RUSSIA
GERMANY
FRANCE SWITZ. ROMANIA
SPAIN ITALY

CANADA

S A

MONGOLIA

5,327
CHINA

SOUTH
KOREA

1,755

TAIWAN

Macao
SAR

Hong Kong
SAR

INDIA

THAILAND

VIETNAM

PHILIPPINES

MALAYSIA

SINGAPORE

INDONESIA

AUSTRALIA

NEW
ZEALAND

SOUTH
AFRICA

Since 2007, new
International Health
Regulations have
provided improved
systems for
responding to
pandemics.

deaths: 774
9.6%

SARS
Case first reported
November 2002 – July 2003

November 2002

February 2003

March 2003

April 2003

May 2003

local transmission occurred

1,000 or more cases
(number given)

total cases reported:
8,096

DEATH RATE
of SARS
2002–03

status of avian influenza pandemic alert in October 2007

Phase 3	Phase 4	Phase 5	Phase 6
No, or very limited, human-to-human transmission	Evidence of increased human-to-human transmission	Evidence of significant human-to-human transmission	Efficient and sustained human-to-human transmission
PANDEMIC ALERT			**PANDEMIC**
New virus causes human cases			

The emergence and spread of resistance to drugs previously effective against infectious diseases threatens the ability to treat infections and save lives.

Bacteria, viruses and parasites cause a wide range of potentially fatal infectious diseases. Antimicrobial drugs include antibiotics, antivirals and medicines active against parasites. These are essential in the management of respiratory infections, diarrhoeal diseases, HIV/AIDS, tuberculosis, STIs and many other infections.

Drug resistance can develop naturally, but it can be made worse by drug misuse, such as improper prescribing or self-prescribing, failure to complete the full course of drugs, the sale of drugs by untrained providers, and counterfeit or poor-quality medications.

Chloroquine-resistant *Plasmodium falciparum* malaria spread rapidly around the globe in the 1980s. Emerging epidemics of healthcare-acquired infections such as MRSA (methicillin-resistant *Staphylococcus aureus*) are increasing problems in hospitals and the community. In developing countries, people are unlikely to have access to expensive alternative treatments.

Actions needed to respond to drug resistance include disease prevention, which reduces the need for drugs and lowers the likelihood that resistant strains will emerge, and full access to, and appropriate use of, antimicrobials. It also includes up-to-date lists of effective drugs and prescribing guidelines, continuing education of healthcare users and providers, and surveillance of infectious diseases and drug resistance. Infection-control practices in healthcare facilities, including hand washing, are essential in preventing infections.

Research is needed to find effective interventions for improving drug use by patients, and drug prescribing and dispensing by healthcare providers.

MULTI-DRUG-RESISTANT TB

Number of laboratory-confirmed cases of MDR tuberculosis
2005

■ 2,000 – 6,600	100 – 249
■ 500 – 999	fewer than 100
■ 250 – 499	none or no data

10% or more of population tested positive to methicillin-resistant *Staphylococcus aureus* (MRSA) *latest available data since 1998*

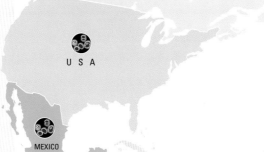

CANADA

USA

MEXICO

GUATEMALA
EL SALVADOR
NICARAGUA
COSTA RICA
PANAMA

○ MONTSERRAT
○ ST VINCENT & GRENADINES
○ TRINIDAD & TOBAGO

VENEZUELA
SURINAME
COLOMBIA
ECUADOR

PERU

BRAZIL

BOLIVIA

PARAGUAY

CHILE   ARGENTINA

CHLOROQUINE–RESISTANT MALARIA

Spread of chloroquine-resistant *Plasmodium falciparum* parasite
1957–1980s

⬭   epicentres of resistance

▓   areas affected

➚ **1960s**   route and date by which it spread

Respiratory Diseases 56–57; Sexually Transmitted Infections 62–63; HIV/AIDS 64–65; Tuberculosis 66–67; Malaria 68–69

ANTIMICROBIAL RESISTANCE

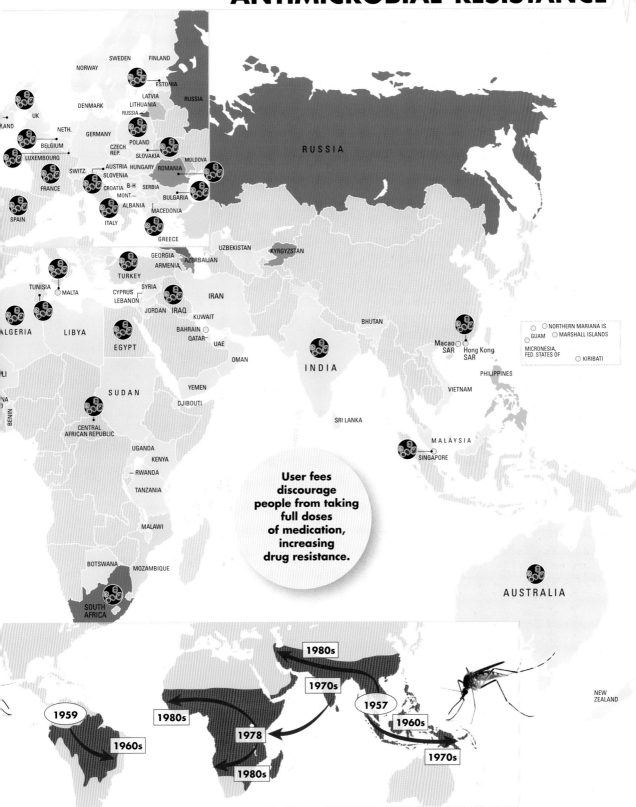

User fees discourage people from taking full doses of medication, increasing drug resistance.

Disability, poor health and poverty are interconnected.

Malnutrition, unsafe living and working conditions, and the limited health services experienced by those living in poverty can all lead to disability; and when disabled people face barriers to participation in education, work and social activities, disability can in turn cause poverty.

Surveys and censuses take very different approaches to measuring disability. Marked differences in the definitions, concepts and methods used to identify people with disabilities make comparing prevalence rates of disability across countries difficult. Best estimates suggest that approximately one person in ten has a disability.

The medical model of disability sees it as a problem of the person, directly caused by disease or trauma that requires medical care. Management of the disability is aimed at cure, or at the individual's adjustment and behaviour change. Categories of disability include physical, sensory, cognitive, intellectual impairments and mental health problems.

The social model sees disability as a complex collection of conditions, many of which are created by the social environment. Management requires social action, and the collective responsibility of society to make the environmental modifications necessary for the full participation of people with disabilities in all areas of social life. Enabling is a human rights issue.

The International Classification of Functioning, Disability and Health (ICF) combines biological, individual and social perspectives of health and disability.

Prevention of disabilities means preventing the causes of disability. Rehabilitation and support services are essential to enable people with disabilities to reach and sustain optimal levels of independence and functioning.

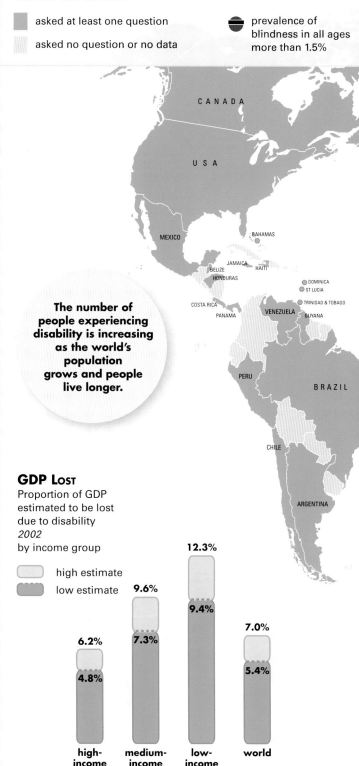

COLLECTING THE DATA
Countries that asked questions on disability in censuses between 1995 and 2004

- asked at least one question
- asked no question or no data
- prevalence of blindness in all ages more than 1.5%

The number of people experiencing disability is increasing as the world's population grows and people live longer.

GDP LOST
Proportion of GDP estimated to be lost due to disability
2002
by income group

- high estimate
- low estimate

	high-income	medium-income	low-income	world
high estimate	6.2%	9.6%	12.3%	7.0%
low estimate	4.8%	7.3%	9.4%	5.4%

Food and Nutrition 28–29; Heart Disease and Stroke 46–47; Injury 54–55; War 76–77

DISABILITY

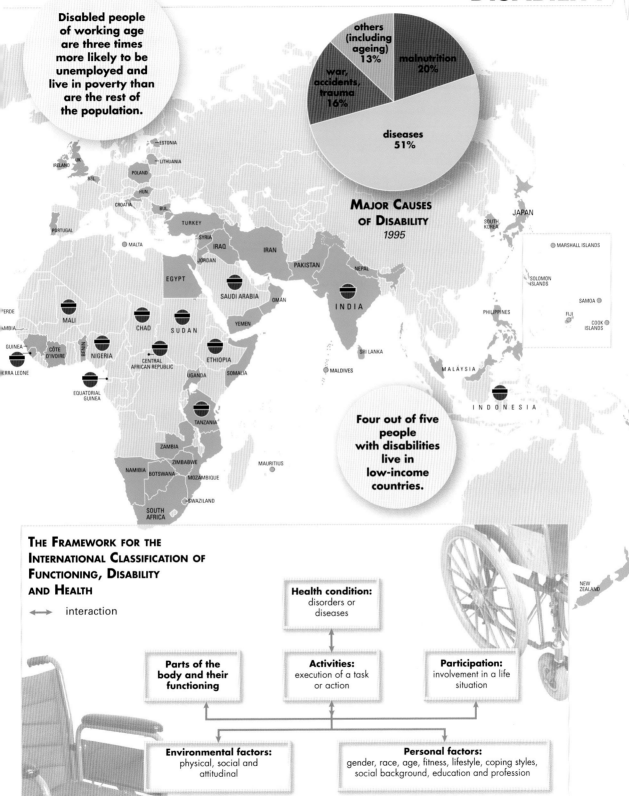

Disabled people of working age are three times more likely to be unemployed and live in poverty than are the rest of the population.

MAJOR CAUSES OF DISABILITY
1995

others (including ageing) 13%

malnutrition 20%

war, accidents, trauma 16%

diseases 51%

Four out of five people with disabilities live in low-income countries.

THE FRAMEWORK FOR THE INTERNATIONAL CLASSIFICATION OF FUNCTIONING, DISABILITY AND HEALTH

⟷ interaction

Health condition: disorders or diseases

Parts of the body and their functioning

Activities: execution of a task or action

Participation: involvement in a life situation

Environmental factors: physical, social and attitudinal

Personal factors: gender, race, age, fitness, lifestyle, coping styles, social background, education and profession

People in all parts of the world are living longer than ever before.

Between 2000 and 2050 the number of children is projected to decline, due to a reduction in birth rates, while the number of people aged 80 and over will increase five-fold, due to improvements in housing, water, nutrition and healthcare. Most of the increase will be in developing countries, where most will live in poverty. The majority of older people are women.

This increase in life expectancy is leading to a decreasing ratio between working-age people and older people. This and other social changes mean there are fewer family members available to look after older people who require care. Increases in age-related disease, disabilities and dementia will put greater demands on healthcare services.

Sustaining good health is essential for older people to continue to be independent and active in family and community life. Health promotion and disease-prevention activities, including maintaining good nutrition and screening for disease, can prevent or delay the onset of non-communicable and chronic diseases such as cancers, heart disease, and stroke.

Older people may have multiple health problems at the same time, and are more likely to die from chronic and degenerative conditions. When older people become unwell, primary healthcare services should provide accessible, integrated care, with monitoring to identify and minimize the development of disabilities. This care is best provided in community-based settings.

POTENTIAL SUPPORT RATIO
Number of people aged 15 to 64 years per person aged 65 years or above
1950–2050 projected

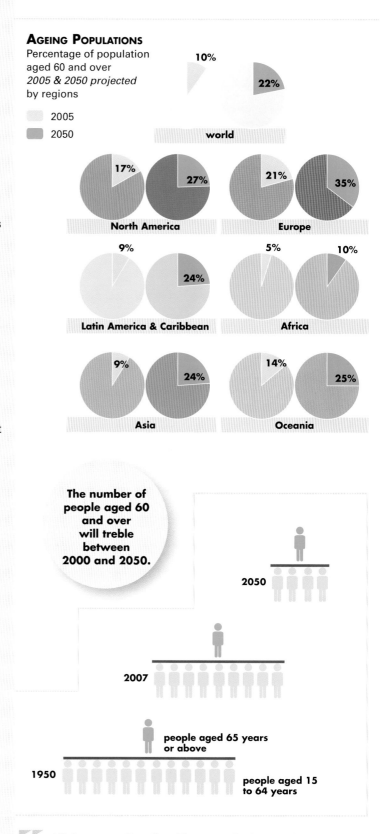

AGEING POPULATIONS
Percentage of population aged 60 and over
2005 & 2050 projected
by regions

2005
2050

10%
22%
world

17% 27%
North America

21% 35%
Europe

9% 24%
Latin America & Caribbean

5% 10%
Africa

9% 24%
Asia

14% 25%
Oceania

The number of people aged 60 and over will treble between 2000 and 2050.

2050

2007

1950

people aged 65 years or above

people aged 15 to 64 years

Life Expectancy 16–17; Heart Disease and Stroke 46–47; Disability 82–83

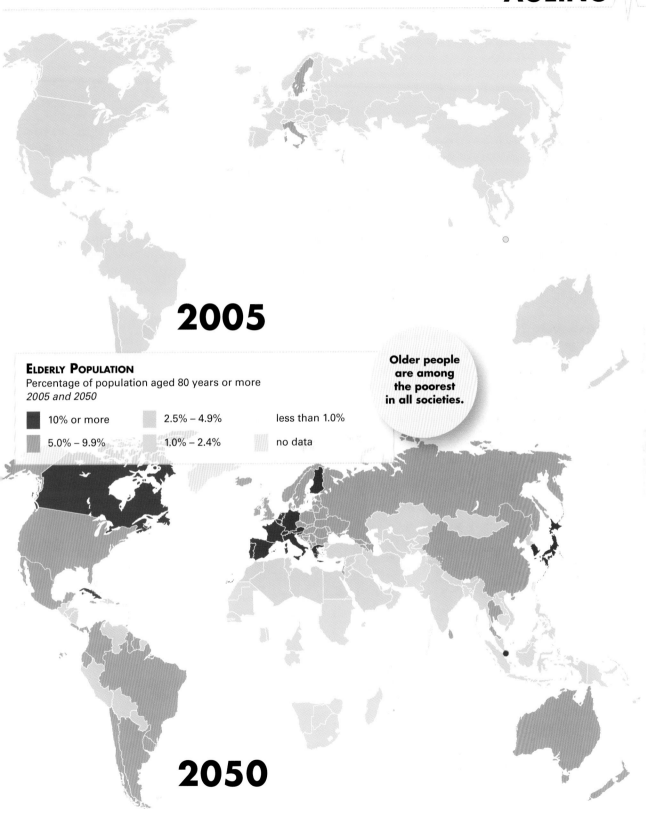

2005

Elderly Population
Percentage of population aged 80 years or more
2005 and 2050

- 10% or more
- 5.0% – 9.9%
- 2.5% – 4.9%
- 1.0% – 2.4%
- less than 1.0%
- no data

Older people are among the poorest in all societies.

2050

Preventing food shortages and enabling people to make healthier dietary choices are both challenges for the 21st century.

Good nutrition is essential for learning. It empowers people by improving their intellectual capacity and their opportunity to generate income, enabling them to lift themselves out of poverty. It is therefore essential for sustainable development. Well-nourished people produce more food; agriculture and nutrition in a population are interdependent.

The World Food Summit of 1996 called for the number of chronically undernourished people to be halved by 2015, but very little progress has been made towards that target.

Overnutrition and obesity are also a cause of concern in developed, and increasingly in developing, countries. Diets high in saturated fat, salt and sugar contribute to the development of chronic diseases, including heart disease and diabetes. Urbanization and the globalization of the food chain are leading to a rapid transition to a high-fat, high-sugar diet, which is having a marked effect on disease patterns.

Illness caused by infectious or toxic agents that enter the body through food is also a major cause of morbidity and mortality, especially in the very young, the elderly, and people whose immune systems are not working well. Increases in foodborne infections such as *Salmonella* and *Campylobacter*, and in chemical contamination of food, have been reported in many countries. Food-safety research is essential to address changes in global production, processing, distribution, and preparation of food.

OVERWEIGHT CHILDREN
Percentage of children aged 5 to 17 years with body mass index >25
2000

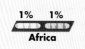 boys
girls

UNDERWEIGHT CHILDREN
Percentage of under-fives who are underweight for their age
latest available data 1996–2004

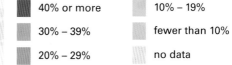

40% or more
30% – 39%
20% – 29%
10% – 19%
fewer than 10%
no data

● problems with food supply or access to it
2007

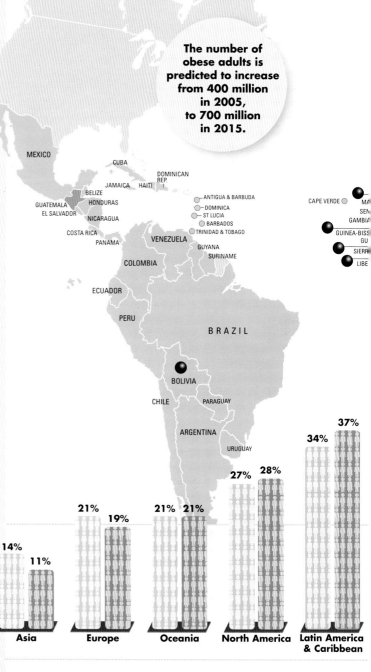

The number of obese adults is predicted to increase from 400 million in 2005, to 700 million in 2015.

1% 1%
Africa

14%
11%
Asia

21%
19%
Europe

21% 21%
Oceania

27% 28%
North America

34% 37%
Latin America & Caribbean

Food and Nutrition 28–29; Heart Disease and Stroke 46–47; Diabetes 48–49; Diarrhoeal Diseases 58–59; Urbanization 72–73

UNHEALTHY DIETS

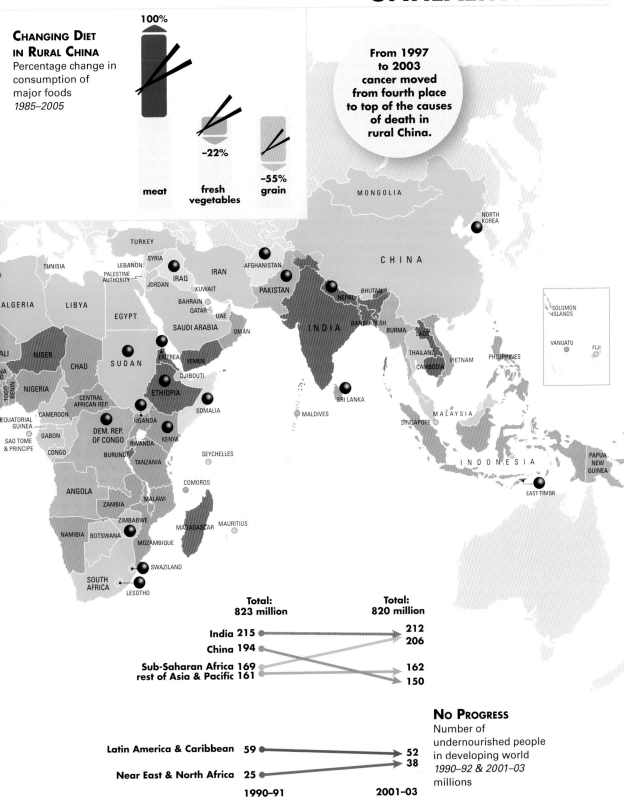

CHANGING DIET IN RURAL CHINA
Percentage change in consumption of major foods
1985–2005

100%

−22%
meat fresh vegetables

−55%
grain

From 1997 to 2003 cancer moved from fourth place to top of the causes of death in rural China.

MONGOLIA

NORTH KOREA

TURKEY

SYRIA
LEBANON
PALESTINE AUTHORITY
JORDAN
IRAQ
IRAN
AFGHANISTAN
KUWAIT
PAKISTAN
BAHRAIN
QATAR
UAE
SAUDI ARABIA
OMAN
TUNISIA
ALGERIA
LIBYA
EGYPT
MALI
NIGER
CHAD
SUDAN
ERITREA
YEMEN
DJIBOUTI
ETHIOPIA
SOMALIA
NIGERIA
BENIN
TOGO
CENTRAL AFRICAN REP.
CAMEROON
EQUATORIAL GUINEA
GABON
SAO TOME & PRINCIPE
CONGO
DEM. REP. OF CONGO
UGANDA
RWANDA
BURUNDI
KENYA
TANZANIA
ANGOLA
ZAMBIA
MALAWI
ZIMBABWE
NAMIBIA
BOTSWANA
MOZAMBIQUE
MADAGASCAR
MAURITIUS
SWAZILAND
SOUTH AFRICA
LESOTHO
SEYCHELLES
COMOROS

CHINA
NEPAL
BHUTAN
INDIA
BANGLADESH
BURMA
LAOS
THAILAND
CAMBODIA
VIETNAM
PHILIPPINES
SRI LANKA
MALDIVES
MALAYSIA
SINGAPORE
INDONESIA
PAPUA NEW GUINEA
EAST TIMOR

SOLOMON ISLANDS
VANUATU
FIJI

Total: 823 million

Total: 820 million

India 215 → 212
China 194 → 206
Sub-Saharan Africa 169 → 162
rest of Asia & Pacific 161 → 150

NO PROGRESS
Number of undernourished people in developing world
1990–92 & 2001–03
millions

Latin America & Caribbean 59 → 52
Near East & North Africa 25 → 38

1990–91   2001–03

The huge shortage of health workers is a global crisis.

Virtually every country has not enough nurses, doctors and other healthcare staff, but the shortage is most acute in the poorest countries, where health systems are weakest. New interventions and technologies, such as anti-retroviral therapy for HIV/AIDS and new vaccine programmes, can only be implemented where there is a sufficiently large, skilled workforce in place.

In most countries, health workers tend to migrate to cities, but global migration of health workers from poor countries with high mortality to wealthier, lower-mortality countries results in the loss of nurses and doctors in countries that can least afford it.

In the countries worst affected by HIV/AIDS, the workload of health workers is increased by the disease, their morale is weakened by lack of resources to deal with it, and they are exposed to infection.

There has been chronic underinvestment in human resources for health, particularly in poor countries where economic reforms have restricted the development of the public health sector. This has led to frozen salaries and recruitment, and poorly resourced facilities. The shortage of health workers is most severe in the poorest rural districts, where there are few incentives and supports in place to attract and retain staff.

HEALTHCARE STAFF

Number of nurses
per 10,000 people
2004 or latest available data

- fewer than 5
- 5 – 9
- 10 – 19
- 20 – 49
- 50 – 99
- 100 or more
- no data

only one doctor
for more than
10,000 people
2004

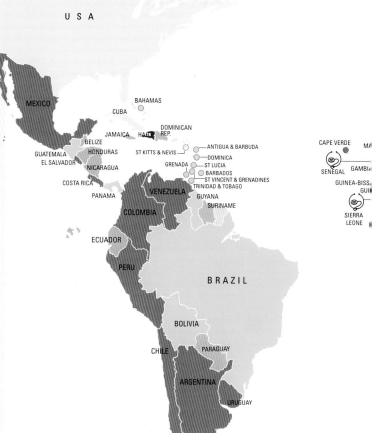

BRAIN DRAIN
Percentage of doctors
trained abroad
latest available data
selected countries

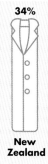

New Zealand	UK	USA	Canada	Australia	Finland	France	Germany
34%	33%	27%	23%	21%	9%	6%	6%

Maternal Health 18–19; Poverty 24–25; Healthcare 36–37;
Vaccine-Preventable Diseases 60–61; HIV/AIDS 64–65

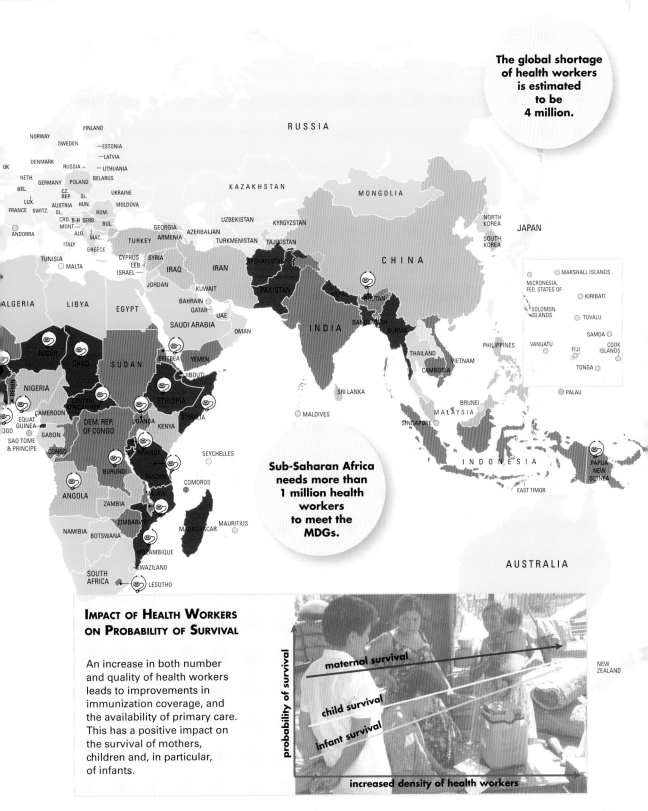

The global shortage of health workers is estimated to be 4 million.

Sub-Saharan Africa needs more than 1 million health workers to meet the MDGs.

IMPACT OF HEALTH WORKERS ON PROBABILITY OF SURVIVAL

An increase in both number and quality of health workers leads to improvements in immunization coverage, and the availability of primary care. This has a positive impact on the survival of mothers, children and, in particular, of infants.

probability of survival

maternal survival

child survival

infant survival

increased density of health workers

Research is essential for health, health equity and economic development.

In 1990, the Commission on Health Research for Development estimated that less than 10 percent of the world's health research resources was spent on the problems of developing countries, whose citizens bore over 90 percent of the global burden of disease: this is known as "the 10/90 gap".

Health research is a driving force for development and the fight against poverty. While spending on it has increased dramatically since 1990, most of it is spent by high-income countries in high-income countries, with little investment in research that directly addresses the health problems of poor people in low- and middle-income countries. A target of 2 percent of national health expenditure to be spent on R&D, has been met only by Argentina and Brazil among low- and middle-income countries.

Essential national health research is needed in every country to plan, co-ordinate, monitor and manage health-research resources and activities. As well as addressing the traditional diseases of poverty there is a need for relevant research to address the massive increase in non-communicable disease in low- and middle-income countries, including research on policies, systems and services for different places and settings. In poor countries, the capacity to design, conduct and utilize health research remains very limited, and is compounded by the brain drain of skilled researchers to wealthy countries and to private research institutions.

PUBLISHED RESEARCH
Biomedical publications
1990–2000
per million population

- less than 1
- 1 – 9
- 10 – 99
- 100 – 700
- no data

public funding of R&D for health more than 0.1% of GDP
2003

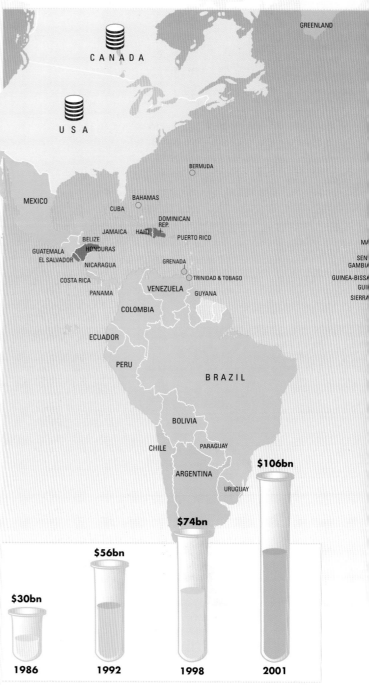

GROWTH OF EXPENDITURE
Global expenditure on health research
1986–2001

$30bn — 1986
$56bn — 1992
$74bn — 1998
$106bn — 2001

HEALTH RESEARCH

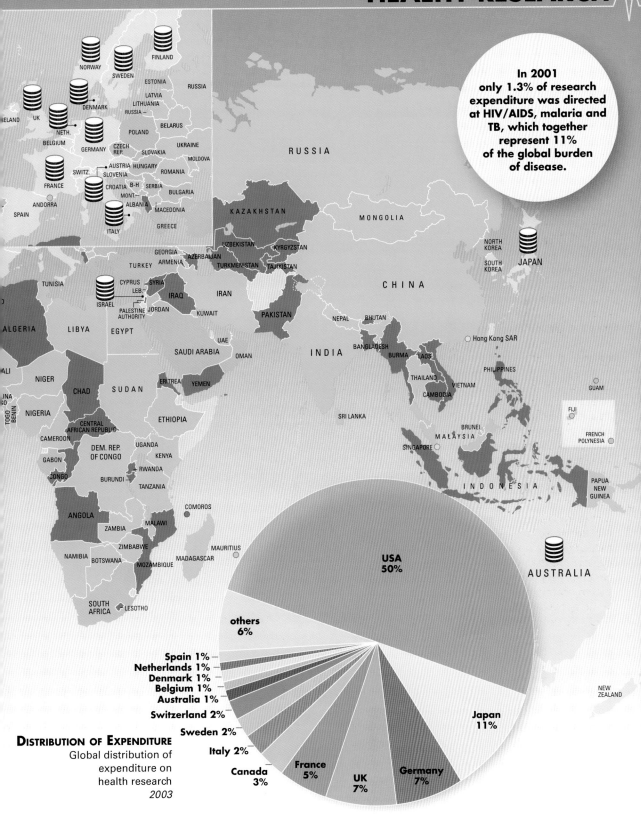

NORWAY
SWEDEN
FINLAND
ESTONIA
RUSSIA
LATVIA
LITHUANIA
RUSSIA
ICELAND
UK
DENMARK
BELARUS
NETH.
POLAND
BELGIUM
GERMANY
UKRAINE
CZECH REP.
SLOVAKIA
MOLDOVA
AUSTRIA HUNGARY
SWITZ.
SLOVENIA
ROMANIA
FRANCE
CROATIA
B-H
SERBIA
BULGARIA
MONT.
ANDORRA
ALBANIA
MACEDONIA
SPAIN
ITALY
GREECE

RUSSIA

MONGOLIA

NORTH KOREA
SOUTH KOREA
JAPAN

KAZAKHSTAN

UZBEKISTAN
KYRGYZSTAN
TURKMENISTAN
TAJIKISTAN

GEORGIA
ARMENIA
AZERBAIJAN

TUNISIA
CYPRUS
LEB.
SYRIA
ISRAEL
PALESTINE AUTHORITY
JORDAN
IRAQ
IRAN
KUWAIT
PAKISTAN

CHINA

NEPAL
BHUTAN

ALGERIA
LIBYA
EGYPT
SAUDI ARABIA
UAE
OMAN
INDIA
BANGLADESH
BURMA
LAOS
Hong Kong SAR

MALI
NIGER
CHAD
SUDAN
ERITREA
YEMEN
THAILAND
VIETNAM
CAMBODIA
PHILIPPINES
GUAM

BURKINA
TOGO
BENIN
NIGERIA
CENTRAL AFRICAN REPUBLIC
ETHIOPIA
SRI LANKA
BRUNEI
MALAYSIA
FIJI
FRENCH POLYNESIA

CAMEROON
GABON
CONGO
DEM. REP. OF CONGO
UGANDA
KENYA
RWANDA
BURUNDI
TANZANIA
SINGAPORE
INDONESIA
PAPUA NEW GUINEA

ANGOLA
ZAMBIA
MALAWI
COMOROS
AUSTRALIA

NAMIBIA
BOTSWANA
ZIMBABWE
MOZAMBIQUE
MADAGASCAR
MAURITIUS

SOUTH AFRICA
LESOTHO

NEW ZEALAND

> In 2001 only 1.3% of research expenditure was directed at HIV/AIDS, malaria and TB, which together represent 11% of the global burden of disease.

Pie chart: DISTRIBUTION OF EXPENDITURE

- USA 50%
- Japan 11%
- Germany 7%
- UK 7%
- France 5%
- Canada 3%
- Italy 2%
- Sweden 2%
- Switzerland 2%
- Australia 1%
- Belgium 1%
- Denmark 1%
- Netherlands 1%
- Spain 1%
- others 6%

DISTRIBUTION OF EXPENDITURE
Global distribution of expenditure on health research
2003

Health and well-being need to be measured in order to provide a clear profile of the distribution of health and disease. This allows for informed decision-making, but it is a complex and difficult procedure.

Health surveillance includes the systematic collection of health-related data, statistical analysis and interpretation, dissemination of this information to those who require it for action, and continuing surveillance to evaluate actions.

Reliable and timely information on health and its determinants are essential to strong health systems. This information is required in order to identify problems and needs, make evidence-based decisions on measures to improve the health of populations, and allocate scarce resources optimally. Unfortunately, health data are most often not available in countries with the greatest need, because of under-investment and a lack of capacity in data collection, analysis and use.

Data on deaths are central for planning health priorities because they indicate the severity of health problems. They are needed to calculate many indicators, from life expectancy to potential years of life lost (PYLLs) and disability adjusted life years (DALYs), used to measure the burden of disease. In many countries not all deaths are registered. Even where all deaths are medically certified, the accuracy of cause-of-death data may be compromised by failure to record all health problems contributing to a person's death, or inappropriate completion of the death certificate.

Huge improvements in health research and information systems are needed to improve health.

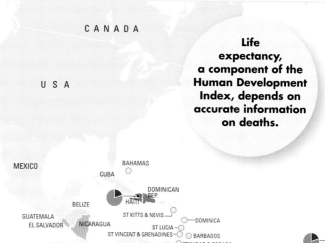

DEATH REGISTRATION
Percentage of deaths registered
2003 or latest available data

- fewer than 25%
- 25% – 49%
- 50% – 74%
- 75% – 99%
- 100%
- no data

YEARS OF LIFE LOST
Cause of more than 80% of premature deaths
2002

- ▶ noncommunicable diseases and injuries
- ◕ communicable diseases

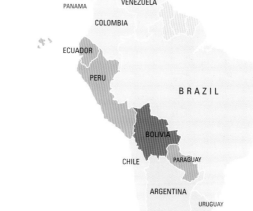

Life expectancy, a component of the Human Development Index, depends on accurate information on deaths.

MEASURING HEALTH

Most deaths are not officially registered.

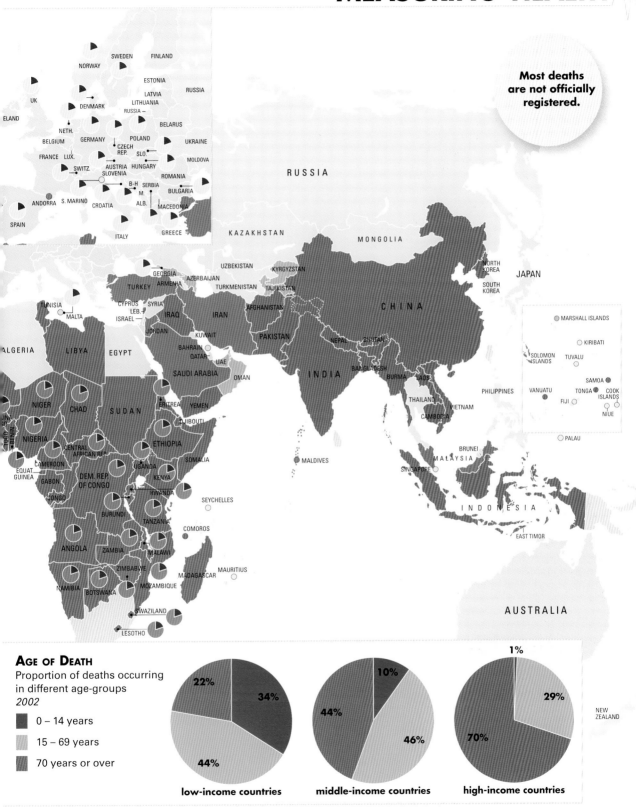

AGE OF DEATH
Proportion of deaths occurring in different age-groups
2002

- 0 – 14 years
- 15 – 69 years
- 70 years or over

low-income countries
- 22%
- 34%
- 44%

middle-income countries
- 10%
- 44%
- 46%

high-income countries
- 1%
- 29%
- 70%

MATERNAL MORTALITY RATIO
Source of data for 2000 estimate

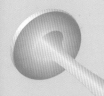

reproductive age-mortality studies 8%

detailed data-gathering to identify the cause of
death of women of reproductive age

**complete vital
registration data 35%**

certification and registration
of individual deaths

**household surveys
or censuses 18%**

the recording of population at
fixed points in time, and interviews
with household members that include
questions about deaths

statistical calculations 39%

calculating the likely number of maternal deaths
from other health data

Total: 173 countries

PART 5

DATES, DEFINITIONS AND DATA

Key scientific discoveries that have influenced our understanding of health and diseases, and the policy changes that have made a difference to the health of populations, are plotted on a timeline overleaf. However, it often takes many years for research findings to be put into practice.

There are many limitations to health statistics. They are only as good as the ability of health information systems to provide data. Many of the poorest countries are those least able to provide accurate information. There is a need for major investment in information systems in order to accurately monitor progress and evaluate the impact of interventions in health and development.

The tables in this section present the main data from the maps in the book, but because of the constraints on its collection, the data need to be interpreted with caution.

1775
Percival Potts describes scrotal cancer in chimney sweeps caused by soot – the first description of occupational exposure to a cancer-causing substance.

1796
Edward Jenner introduces vaccination against smallpox using cowpox virus.

200 BCE
Galen describes the roles of heredity, lifestyle and environment in health.

1670s
Antonie van Leeuwenhoek develops microscope and identifies bacteria.

| 400BCE | 200BCE | 1600 | 1700 | 1750 |

400 BCE
Hippocrates describes the importance of diet, exercise and fresh air for health.

1628
William Harvey describes circulation of blood, pumped by the heart.

1754
James Lind reports trial of treatments for scurvy. Discovery that citrus juice prevents and treats disease improves the lives of sailors and opportunities for long distance trade. It takes until 1795 for British Navy to order general issue of citrus fruit.

1798
Thomas Malthus predicts that population growth will exceed food supply.

1348–50
Plague kills third of population of Western Europe.

1700
Bernardino Ramazzini describes health hazards of various occupations. He also promotes the use of quinine-rich cinchona bark for malaria.

SIGNIFICANT EVENTS IN PUBLIC HEALTH
400BCE–1899

1847
Ignaz Semmelweiss demonstrates that puerperal fever ("childbed fever") is contagious and that its incidence could be drastically reduced by hand-washing among healthcare workers.

1854
In the cholera outbreak in London, John Snow plots the location of cases on a map and relates them to the water supply. Following his advice to remove the handle of the Broad Street pump, the epidemic is contained.

1848
First Public Health Act is passed in England and Wales. Public health becomes the responsibility of local people through boards of health.

1862
Pasteurization, the process of heating liquids to destroy harmful organisms, is described by Louis Pasteur.

1897
Malaria transmission and life-cycle described.

1818
First successful transfusion of human blood.

1800

1850

1900

1842
Edwin Chadwick proves that life expectancy is much lower in towns than in the countryside, leading to improvements in housing, working conditions, and sanitation.

1850
Lemuel Shattuck links environmental and social factors to health, urges social reform and the documentation of vital statistics.

1865
Joseph Lister promotes the concept of sterile surgery, introducing carbolic acid to sterilize instruments and clean wounds.

1848
Rudolf Virchow reports that a cholera outbreak could not be resolved by treating individual patients, and calls for radical changes to promote the health of the entire population.

1860
Florence Nightingale School of Nursing and Midwifery opens.

1890
Koch's postulates describe criteria designed to establish a causal relationship between a microbe and a disease.

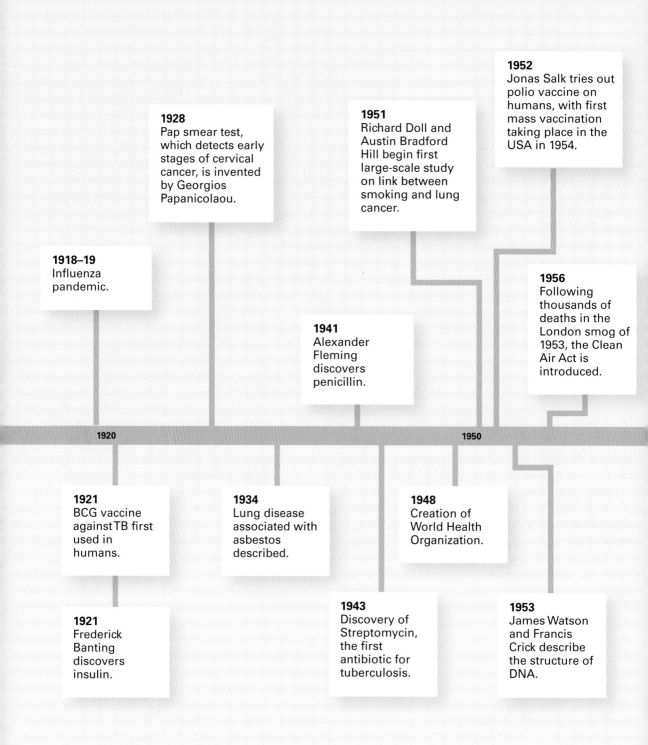

1952
Jonas Salk tries out polio vaccine on humans, with first mass vaccination taking place in the USA in 1954.

1928
Pap smear test, which detects early stages of cervical cancer, is invented by Georgios Papanicolaou.

1951
Richard Doll and Austin Bradford Hill begin first large-scale study on link between smoking and lung cancer.

1918–19
Influenza pandemic.

1941
Alexander Fleming discovers penicillin.

1956
Following thousands of deaths in the London smog of 1953, the Clean Air Act is introduced.

1920

1950

1921
BCG vaccine against TB first used in humans.

1934
Lung disease associated with asbestos described.

1948
Creation of World Health Organization.

1921
Frederick Banting discovers insulin.

1943
Discovery of Streptomycin, the first antibiotic for tuberculosis.

1953
James Watson and Francis Crick describe the structure of DNA.

SIGNIFICANT EVENTS IN PUBLIC HEALTH
1900–2007

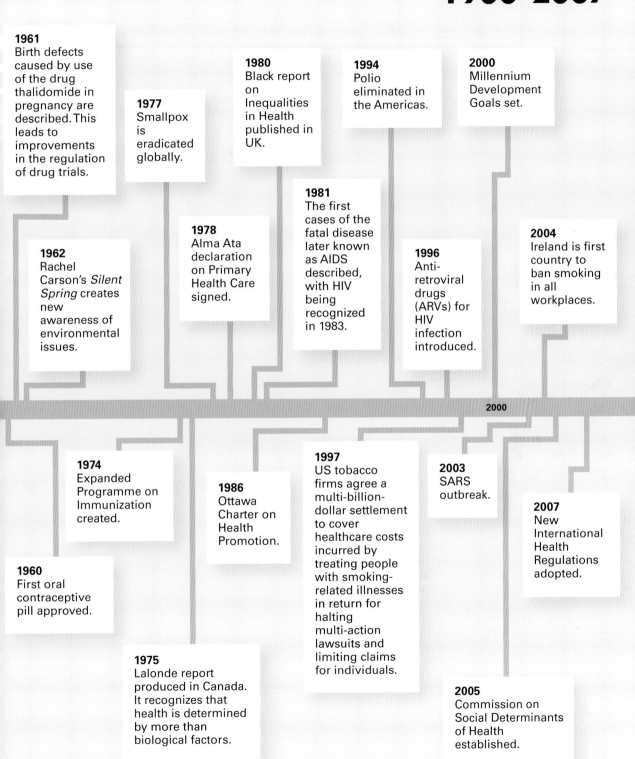

1961
Birth defects caused by use of the drug thalidomide in pregnancy are described. This leads to improvements in the regulation of drug trials.

1977
Smallpox is eradicated globally.

1980
Black report on Inequalities in Health published in UK.

1994
Polio eliminated in the Americas.

2000
Millennium Development Goals set.

1962
Rachel Carson's *Silent Spring* creates new awareness of environmental issues.

1978
Alma Ata declaration on Primary Health Care signed.

1981
The first cases of the fatal disease later known as AIDS described, with HIV being recognized in 1983.

1996
Anti-retroviral drugs (ARVs) for HIV infection introduced.

2004
Ireland is first country to ban smoking in all workplaces.

2000

1974
Expanded Programme on Immunization created.

1986
Ottawa Charter on Health Promotion.

1997
US tobacco firms agree a multi-billion-dollar settlement to cover healthcare costs incurred by treating people with smoking-related illnesses in return for halting multi-action lawsuits and limiting claims for individuals.

2003
SARS outbreak.

2007
New International Health Regulations adopted.

1960
First oral contraceptive pill approved.

1975
Lalonde report produced in Canada. It recognizes that health is determined by more than biological factors.

2005
Commission on Social Determinants of Health established.

GLOSSARY

Access to an improved water source: Having a household connection, or a public standpipe, borehole, protected well or spring or rainwater collection within 1 kilometre of the dwelling that provides at least 20 litres per person per day.

Age-standardized mortality rate: A weighted average of the age-specific mortality rates per 100,000 persons, in which the weights are the proportion of persons in the corresponding age-groups of the WHO standard population.

Acquired Immune Deficiency Syndrome (AIDS): The late clinical stage in infection with the Human Immunodeficiency Virus (HIV).

Acute lower respiratory-tract infection (ALRI): Pneumonia, bronchiolitis and bronchitis. The organisms causing ALRI may be bacteria or viruses.

Anti-retroviral therapy (ART): Drug treatment for HIV/AIDS that uses combinations of anti-retroviral (ARV) drugs to suppress replication of the human immunodeficiency virus (HIV) and stop disease progression.

Body mass index (BMI): A measure, defined as weight in kilograms divided by the square of height in metres, used to determine whether a person is under- or over-weight, or obese.

Carcinogen: a substance or agent that causes cancer.

Cardiovascular disease (CVD): Any disease of the heart or blood vessels, including stroke and high blood pressure.

Chronic obstructive pulmonary disease (COPD): A general term used to describe chronic lung diseases that cause limitations in lung airflow. It includes the conditions known as chronic bronchitis and emphysema.

Dependency ratio: The ratio of economically inactive (children and old people) to economically active in a population. Children are usually defined as those aged under 15, and old people as those aged 65 and over.

Determinant: Any factor, whether event, characteristic or other definable entity, that brings about a change in a health condition or other defined characteristic

Directly observed therapy (DOTS): A patient is watched taking medication to ensure the right combination is taken for the correct duration. Healthcare workers, or family or community members can be involved.

Disability adjusted life years (DALYs): A measure that extends the concept of **potential years of life lost (PYLL)** due to premature death to include equivalent years of "healthy" life lost by virtue of being in a state of poor health or disability. Used to measure the burden of disease on a defined population and the effectiveness of interventions.

Epidemic: The occurrence in a community or region of cases of an illness, specific health-related behaviour, or other health-related events clearly in excess of normal expectancy.

Gross domestic product (GDP): A measure of the production of good and services in an economy, it calculates the total value added by all resident producers in an economy.

Gross national income (GNI): The **gross domestic product** plus income from abroad.

Human Development Index (HDI): An index calculated using indicators representing: longevity (life expectancy at birth); knowledge (adult literacy rate and mean years of schooling); and income (real GDP per capita in purchasing-power-parity dollars).

Human immunodeficiency virus (HIV): The pathogenic organism responsible for **Acquired immunodeficiency syndrome (AIDS)**.

Human papilloma virus (HPV): A virus that can cause abnormal tissue growth and other changes to cells. Infection with certain types of HPV increases the risk of developing cervical cancer.

Human Poverty Index (HPI): An index calculated using indicators representing longevity, knowledge and a decent standard of living. For developing countries the index uses indicators of life expectancy, adult illiteracy, access to safe water, and proportion of undernourished children. There is a separate HPI for developed countries, based on different measures.

Improved sanitation: Adequate facilities for the disposal of human excreta, including connection to a sewer or septic tank system, a pour-flush latrine, a simple pit latrine or a ventilated improved pit latrine. It is considered adequate if it is private or shared (but not public) and if it can effectively prevent human, animal and insect contact with faeces.

Incidence: The number of new cases of a disease in a defined population within a specified period of time.

Inequality ratio: The factor by which the income of the richest sector of a population exceeds that of the poorest sector.

Infant mortality rate (IMR): For every 1,000 live births, the number of babies who die before the age of one.

Insecticide-treated net (ITN): A net, impregnated with insecticide, designed to cover a sleeping person and prevent them from being bitten by mosquitoes and other insects.

International Agency for Research on Cancer (IARC): a World Health Organization agency.

Intergovernmental Panel on Climate Change (IPCC): Established by the World Meteorological Organization (WMO) and the United Nations Environment Programme (UNEP) in 1988 to assess scientific, technical and socio-economic information relevant to the understanding of climate change, its potential impacts and options for adaptation and mitigation.

Life expectancy: Average number of years that a newborn is expected to live if current mortality rates continue to apply.

Maternal death: The death of a woman while pregnant or within 42 days of termination of pregnancy, irrespective of the duration and site of the pregnancy, from any cause related to or aggravated by the pregnancy or its management but not from accidental or incidental causes.

Maternal mortality ratio: Number of **maternal deaths** per 100,000 live births during a specified period, usually a year.

Neonatal death: Within 28 days of birth.

Net enrolment ratio: The ratio of the number of children of official school age who are enrolled in primary school, to the total population of the corresponding official school age.

Oral rehydration therapy (ORT): A cheap and effective orally administered treatment for diarrhoea-related dehydration, consisting of a solution of salts and sugars.

Outbreak: An epidemic limited to localized increase in the incidence of disease, such as in a town or institution.

Pandemic: An epidemic occurring worldwide, or over a very wide area, crossing international boundaries and usually affecting a large number of people.

Perinatal: Around the time of birth, conventionally limited to the period between 28 weeks of gestation and one week after birth.

Potential years of life lost (PYLL): A measure of the relative impact of various diseases and lethal forces on a society, calculated from the number of deaths multiplied by a standard life expectancy at the age at which death occurs.

Prevalence: The number of events, such as instances of a given disease or other condition, in a given population at a given time.

Primary healthcare: Essential healthcare made universally accessible to individuals and families. See www.who.int/topics/primary_health_care/en/ for more detail.

Screening: A health service in which members of a defined population, who do not necessarily perceive they are at risk of a disease or its complications, are asked a question or offered a test, to identify those individuals who are more likely to be helped than harmed by further tests or treatment.

Under-five mortality rate: The probability of a child born in a specific year or period dying before reaching the age of five, if subject to age-specific mortality rates of that period.

Countries	Life expectancy At birth 2005	Maternal deaths Per 100,000 live births 2000	Under-five deaths Per 1,000 live births 2005	Cancer deaths	CVD deaths	Diabetes % of population with condition 2003
				age-standardized mortality rate per 100,000 people 2002		
Afghanistan	47	1,900	257	153	706	8.2%
Albania	74	55	18	154	537	3.8%
Algeria	72	140	39	103	314	4.1%
Angola	41	1,700	260	179	486	2.7%
Antigua and Barbuda	–	–	12	144	343	5.8%
Argentina	75	82	16	142	212	5.4%
Armenia	72	55	29	146	498	8.1%
Australia	81	8	6	127	140	6.2%
Austria	79	4	5	127	204	9.6%
Azerbaijan	67	94	89	113	613	6.9%
Bahamas	71	60	15	112	222	9.0%
Bahrain	75	28	11	127	312	14.9%
Bangladesh	64	380	73	111	428	3.9%
Barbados	76	95	12	135	245	8.5%
Belarus	68	35	9	143	592	6.9%
Belgium	79	10	5	148	162	4.2%
Belize	72	140	17	147	317	5.7%
Benin	55	850	150	154	432	2.1%
Bhutan	64	420	75	112	441	3.7%
Bolivia	65	420	65	256	260	4.8%
Bosnia and Herzegovina	74	31	15	121	492	9.6%
Botswana	34	100	120	124	338	3.6%
Brazil	71	260	33	142	341	5.2%
Brunei	77	37	9	114	210	10.7%
Bulgaria	73	32	15	125	554	10.0%
Burkina Faso	48	1,000	191	162	459	2.7%
Burma	61	360	104	115	432	1.1%
Burundi	44	1,000	190	146	439	1.3%
Cambodia	57	450	143	148	392	2.0%
Cameroon	46	730	149	150	436	0.8%
Canada	80	6	6	138	141	9.0%
Cape Verde	71	150	35	127	356	2.3%
Central African Republic	39	1,100	193	154	445	2.3%
Chad	44	1,100	208	156	443	2.7%
Chile	78	31	10	137	165	5.6%
China	72	56	27	148	291	2.7%
Colombia	73	130	21	117	240	4.3%
Comoros	64	480	71	128	381	2.5%
Congo	53	510	108	134	393	2.6%
Congo, Dem. Rep.	44	990	205	161	465	2.5%
Cook Islands	–	–	20	69	326	6.6%
Costa Rica	78	43	12	125	185	6.9%
Côte d'Ivoire	46	690	196	160	436	2.3%
Croatia	75	8	7	167	356	5.8%
Cuba	78	33	7	129	215	13.2%
Cyprus	79	47	5	94	354	5.1%
Czech Republic	76	9	4	177	315	9.5%
Denmark	78	5	5	167	182	6.9%

HEALTH PROBLEMS

Deaths of under-fives Cause of death as % of all deaths			Measles % of infants receiving dose of vaccine 2005	HIV/AIDS % of people aged 15–49 with HIV 2005	Tuberculosis Number of cases per 100,000 people 2005	Countries
umonia 2000	diarrhoea 2000	malaria 2000				
4.8%	18.9%	1.0%	64%	<0.1	288	Afghanistan
0.6%	10.5%	0.4%	97%	–	28	Albania
3.7%	11.9%	0.5%	83%	0.1%	55	Algeria
4.8%	19.1%	8.3%	45%	3.7%	333	Angola
1.5%	2.4%	0.0%	99%	–	9	Antigua and Barbuda
3.4%	1.3%	0.0%	99%	0.6%	51	Argentina
11.8%	10.5%	0.5%	94%	0.1%	79	Armenia
1.2%	0.1%	0.0%	94%	0.1%	6	Australia
0.7%	0.0%	0.0%	75%	0.3%	9	Austria
8.4%	15.3%	1.0%	98%	0.1%	85	Azerbaijan
5.3%	0.8%	0.0%	85%	3.3%	49	Bahamas
1.4%	0.7%	0.0%	99%	<0.1	43	Bahrain
17.6%	20.0%	0.7%	81%	–	406	Bangladesh
0.0%	0.0%	0.0%	93%	1.5%	12	Barbados
9.0%	1.5%	0.0%	99%	0.3%	70	Belarus
0.8%	0.3%	0.0%	88%	0.3%	10	Belgium
6.9%	3.5%	0.0%	95%	2.5%	55	Belize
21.1%	17.1%	27.2%	85%	1.8%	144	Benin
8.8%	20.9%	0.8%	93%	<0.1	174	Bhutan
17.1%	14.3%	0.7%	64%	0.1%	280	Bolivia
2.5%	0.6%	0.0%	90%	<0.1	57	Bosnia and Herzegovina
1.4%	1.1%	0.0%	90%	24.1%	556	Botswana
3.2%	12.0%	0.5%	99%	0.5%	76	Brazil
0.7%	1.1%	0.0%	97%	<0.1	63	Brunei
6.1%	2.3%	0.0%	96%	<0.1	41	Bulgaria
23.3%	18.8%	20.3%	84%	2.0%	461	Burkina Faso
19.3%	21.1%	9.0%	72%	1.3%	170	Burma
22.8%	18.2%	8.4%	75%	3.3%	602	Burundi
20.6%	16.6%	0.9%	79%	1.6%	703	Cambodia
21.5%	17.3%	22.8%	68%	5.4%	206	Cameroon
1.1%	0.2%	0.0%	94%	0.3%	4	Canada
3.3%	12.2%	4.3%	65%	–	327	Cape Verde
8.7%	14.7%	18.5%	35%	10.7%	483	Central African Republic
22.8%	18.1%	22.3%	23%	3.5%	495	Chad
6.2%	0.5%	0.0%	90%	0.3%	16	Chile
13.4%	11.8%	0.4%	86%	0.1%	208	China
10.4%	10.3%	0.2%	89%	0.6%	66	Colombia
16.3%	13.6%	19.4%	80%	<0.1	89	Comoros
13.6%	11.2%	25.7%	56%	5.3%	449	Congo
23.1%	18.1%	16.9%	70%	3.2%	541	Congo, Dem. Rep.
1.1%	0.7%	0.0%	99%	–	26	Cook Islands
4.0%	3.0%	0.0%	89%	0.3%	17	Costa Rica
19.6%	14.8%	20.5%	51%	7.1%	659	Côte d'Ivoire
1.3%	0.3%	0.0%	96%	<0.1	65	Croatia
4.1%	1.3%	0.0%	98%	0.1%	11	Cuba
1.7%	3.2%	0.0%	86%	–	5	Cyprus
3.6%	0.2%	0.0%	97%	0.1%	11	Czech Republic
0.9%	0.3%	0.0%	95%	0.2%	6	Denmark

Countries	Life expectancy At birth 2005	Maternal deaths Per 100,000 live births 2000	Under-five deaths Per 1,000 live births 2005	Cancer deaths	CVD deaths	Diabetes % of population with condition 2003
				age-standardized mortality rate per 100,000 people 2002		
Djibouti	53	730	133	116	533	4.9%
Dominica	–	–	15	144	257	8.4%
Dominican Republic	68	150	31	131	381	10.0%
East Timor	56	660	61	118	441	1.4%
Ecuador	75	130	25	129	244	4.8%
Egypt	70	84	33	84	560	9.8%
El Salvador	71	150	27	102	223	6.2%
Equatorial Guinea	42	880	205	155	438	2.5%
Eritrea	55	630	78	133	398	1.9%
Estonia	72	63	7	150	435	9.7%
Ethiopia	48	850	164	147	435	1.9%
Fiji	68	75	18	86	470	8.3%
Finland	79	6	4	115	201	7.2%
France	80	17	5	142	118	6.2%
Gabon	54	420	91	158	410	2.9%
Gambia	57	540	137	144	413	2.2%
Georgia	71	32	45	91	584	9.0%
Germany	79	8	5	141	211	10.2%
Ghana	57	540	112	138	404	3.3%
Greece	78	9	5	132	258	6.1%
Grenada	–	–	21	199	448	6.8%
Guatemala	68	240	43	93	188	5.5%
Guinea	54	740	150	156	432	2.0%
Guinea-Bissau	45	1,100	200	159	449	2.0%
Guyana	64	170	63	86	526	6.0%
Haiti	52	680	120	112	402	5.7%
Honduras	68	110	40	139	348	5.7%
Hungary	73	16	8	201	364	9.7%
Iceland	81	0	3	136	164	2.0%
India	64	540	74	109	428	5.9%
Indonesia	68	230	36	132	361	1.9%
Iran	71	76	36	113	466	3.6%
Iraq	60	250	125	112	508	7.7%
Ireland	78	5	5	151	214	3.4%
Israel	80	17	5	133	136	7.1%
Italy	80	5	4	134	174	6.6%
Jamaica	71	87	20	151	326	7.2%
Japan	82	10	4	119	106	6.9%
Jordan	72	41	26	144	384	7.0%
Kazakhstan	64	210	31	167	713	5.5%
Kenya	48	1,000	120	139	401	2.5%
Kiribati	–	–	65	52	273	6.2%
Korea, North	64	67	55	102	371	5.2%
Korea, South	78	20	6	169	186	6.4%
Kuwait	77	5	12	78	309	12.8%
Kyrgyzstan	67	110	67	106	602	4.3%
Laos	55	650	79	150	476	1.1%
Latvia	72	42	10	156	482	9.9%

HEALTH PROBLEMS

Deaths of under-fives Cause of death as % of all deaths			Measles % of infants receiving dose of vaccine	HIV/AIDS % of people aged 15–49 with HIV	Tuberculosis Number of cases per 100,000 people	Countries
pneumonia 2000	diarrhoea 2000	malaria 2000	2005	2005	2005	
20.4%	16.6%	0.8%	65%	3.1%	1,161	Djibouti
0.0%	0.0%	0.0%	98%	–	24	Dominica
13.0%	11.7%	0.6%	99%	1.1%	116	Dominican Republic
19.6%	21.9%	0.4%	48%	–	713	East Timor
12.0%	11.0%	0.5%	93%	0.3%	202	Ecuador
14.6%	12.8%	0.4%	98%	<0.1	32	Egypt
13.4%	12.4%	0.5%	99%	–	68	El Salvador
17.3%	13.6%	24.0%	51%	3.2%	355	Equatorial Guinea
18.6%	15.6%	13.6%	84%	2.4%	515	Eritrea
2.1%	1.4%	0.0%	96%	1.3%	46	Estonia
22.3%	17.3%	6.1%	59%	–	546	Ethiopia
9.2%	10.6%	0.0%	70%	0.1%	30	Fiji
1.2%	0.8%	0.0%	97%	0.1%	5	Finland
0.6%	0.9%	0.0%	87%	0.4%	10	France
10.7%	8.8%	28.3%	55%	7.9%	385	Gabon
15.5%	12.2%	29.4%	84%	2.4%	352	Gambia
12.5%	11.5%	0.3%	92%	0.2%	86	Georgia
0.7%	0.2%	0.0%	93%	0.1%	6	Germany
14.6%	12.2%	33.0%	83%	2.3%	380	Ghana
2.6%	0.0%	0.0%	88%	0.2%	15	Greece
9.5%	1.6%	0.0%	99%	–	8	Grenada
15.0%	13.1%	0.4%	77%	0.9%	110	Guatemala
20.9%	16.5%	24.5%	59%	1.5%	431	Guinea
23.4%	18.6%	21.0%	80%	3.8%	293	Guinea-Bissau
5.2%	21.4%	0.7%	92%	2.4%	194	Guyana
20.2%	16.5%	0.7%	54%	3.8%	405	Haiti
13.8%	12.2%	0.4%	92%	1.5%	99	Honduras
3.9%	0.1%	0.0%	99%	0.1%	25	Hungary
0.0%	0.0%	0.0%	90%	0.2%	2	Iceland
18.5%	20.3%	0.9%	58%	0.9%	299	India
14.4%	18.3%	0.5%	72%	0.1%	262	Indonesia
6.4%	5.5%	0.2%	94%	0.2%	30	Iran
17.6%	13.2%	0.7%	90%	–	76	Iraq
1.3%	0.0%	0.0%	84%	0.2%	10	Ireland
0.4%	0.6%	0.0%	95%	–	6	Israel
1.0%	0.0%	0.0%	87%	0.5%	5	Italy
9.3%	9.6%	0.0%	84%	1.5%	10	Jamaica
3.9%	0.4%	0.0%	99%	<0.1	38	Japan
11.7%	10.7%	0.3%	95%	–	6	Jordan
16.9%	14.5%	0.8%	99%	0.1%	155	Kazakhstan
19.9%	16.5%	13.6%	69%	6.1%	936	Kenya
11.5%	21.9%	0.7%	56%	–	426	Kiribati
15.2%	18.9%	0.7%	96%	–	179	Korea, North
1.8%	0.4%	0.0%	99%	<0.1	135	Korea, South
4.4%	0.7%	0.0%	99%	–	28	Kuwait
16.7%	14.1%	0.9%	99%	0.1%	133	Kyrgyzstan
19.1%	15.6%	0.7%	41%	0.1%	306	Laos
1.2%	0.0%	0.0%	95%	0.8%	66	Latvia

Countries	Life expectancy At birth 2005	Maternal deaths Per 100,000 live births 2000	Under-five deaths Per 1,000 live births 2005	Cancer deaths	CVD deaths	Diabetes % of population with condition 2003
				age-standardized mortality rate per 100,000 people 2002		
Lebanon	72	150	30	90	453	6.4%
Lesotho	34	550	132	139	404	3.1%
Liberia	42	760	235	169	485	2.0%
Libya	74	97	19	79	411	3.7%
Lithuania	73	13	9	161	391	9.4%
Luxembourg	79	28	5	134	177	3.8%
Macedonia	74	23	17	145	504	4.9%
Madagascar	56	550	119	147	430	2.5%
Malawi	40	1,800	125	150	430	1.7%
Malaysia	74	41	12	139	274	9.4%
Maldives	67	110	42	123	484	1.8%
Mali	48	1,200	218	166	456	2.0%
Malta	79	0	6	124	214	9.2%
Marshall Islands	–	–	58	125	526	8.6%
Mauritania	53	100	125	158	451	3.5%
Mauritius	73	24	15	79	434	10.7%
Mexico	76	83	27	88	163	7.4%
Micronesia, Fed. Sts.	68	–	42	93	410	6.7%
Moldova	69	36	16	116	619	9.3%
Mongolia	65	110	49	306	488	1.4%
Montenegro*	74	–	10	149	508	5.6%
Morocco	70	220	40	67	411	4.2%
Mozambique	42	1,000	145	124	371	3.1%
Namibia	46	300	62	146	385	3.1%
Nauru	–	–	30	138	666	30.2%
Nepal	62	740	74	118	436	4.1%
Netherlands	79	16	5	155	171	3.7%
New Zealand	79	7	6	139	175	7.6%
Nicaragua	70	230	37	120	305	6.1%
Niger	45	1,600	256	169	456	3.1%
Nigeria	44	800	194	157	452	2.2%
Niue	–	–	38	74	339	6.8%
Norway	80	16	4	137	181	6.7%
Oman	75	87	12	105	409	11.4%
Pakistan	64	500	100	107	425	8.5%
Palau	–	–	11	92	396	8.7%
Palestine Authority	73	100	–	–	–	7.4%
Panama	75	160	24	108	182	7.3%
Papua New Guinea	56	300	74	118	442	1.9%
Paraguay	71	170	23	141	291	3.9%
Peru	71	410	27	175	190	5.1%
Philippines	71	200	33	91	336	2.4%
Poland	75	13	8	180	324	9.0%
Portugal	78	5	5	140	208	7.8%
Puerto Rico	–	–	–	–	–	13.2%
Qatar	73	140	12	75	340	16.0%
Romania	72	49	19	141	479	9.3%
Russia	65	67	14	152	688	9.2%

HEALTH PROBLEMS

Deaths of under-fives Cause of death as % of all deaths			Measles % of infants receiving dose of vaccine 2005	HIV/AIDS % of people aged 15–49 with HIV 2005	Tuberculosis Number of cases per 100,000 people 2005	Countries
pneumonia 2000	diarrhoea 2000	malaria 2000				
1.1%	1.0%	0.0%	96%	0.1%	12	Lebanon
4.7%	3.9%	0.0%	85%	23.2%	588	Lesotho
23.0%	17.3%	18.9%	94%	–	507	Liberia
8.5%	8.4%	0.0%	97%	–	18	Libya
5.3%	0.3%	0.0%	97%	0.2%	63	Lithuania
1.1%	0.0%	0.0%	95%	0.2%	9	Luxembourg
4.3%	5.0%	0.0%	96%	<0.1	33	Macedonia
20.7%	16.9%	20.1%	59%	0.5%	396	Madagascar
22.6%	18.1%	14.1%	82%	14.1%	518	Malawi
4.0%	5.4%	0.1%	90%	0.5%	131	Malaysia
17.5%	20.3%	0.6%	97%	–	53	Maldives
23.9%	18.3%	16.9%	86%	1.7%	578	Mali
0.0%	0.0%	0.0%	86%	0.1%	4	Malta
13.5%	14.1%	0.0%	86%	–	269	Marshall Islands
22.3%	16.2%	12.2%	61%	0.7%	590	Mauritania
3.9%	1.2%	0.0%	98%	0.6%	132	Mauritius
8.5%	5.1%	0.0%	96%	0.3%	27	Mexico
11.3%	8.0%	0.0%	96%	–	123	Micronesia, Fed. Sts.
15.5%	2.0%	0.0%	97%	1.1%	149	Moldova
17.1%	14.5%	1.0%	99%	<0.1	206	Mongolia
9.1%	6.0%	0.0%	96%	0.2%	42	Montenegro*
14.0%	12.2%	0.4%	97%	0.1%	73	Morocco
21.2%	16.5%	18.9%	77%	16.1%	597	Mozambique
3.0%	2.5%	0.0%	73%	19.6%	577	Namibia
30.3%	37.8%	0.0%	80%	–	156	Nauru
18.5%	20.5%	0.8%	74%	0.5%	244	Nepal
1.1%	0.0%	0.0%	96%	0.2%	5	Netherlands
2.7%	0.2%	0.0%	82%	0.1%	9	New Zealand
13.7%	12.2%	0.4%	96%	0.2%	74	Nicaragua
25.1%	19.8%	14.3%	83%	1.1%	294	Niger
20.1%	15.7%	24.1%	35%	3.9%	536	Nigeria
–	–	–	99%	–	87	Niue
1.4%	0.3%	0.0%	90%	0.1%	4	Norway
7.2%	8.1%	0.1%	98%	–	11	Oman
19.3%	14.0%	0.7%	78%	0.1%	297	Pakistan
12.4%	9.7%	0.0%	98%		61	Palau
–	–	–	–	–	–	Palestine Authority
10.8%	10.7%	0.2%	99%	0.9%	46	Panama
18.5%	15.3%	0.8%	60%	1.8%	475	Papua New Guinea
11.9%	10.7%	0.3%	90%	0.4%	100	Paraguay
13.6%	12.2%	0.4%	80%	0.6%	206	Peru
13.4%	12.0%	0.4%	80%	<0.1	450	Philippines
2.7%	0.1%	0.0%	98%	0.1%	29	Poland
1.8%	0.1%	0.1%	93%	0.4%	25	Portugal
–	–	–	–	–	–	Puerto Rico
7.7%	8.4%	0.0%	99%	–	65	Qatar
27.1%	2.5%	0.0%	97%	<0.1	146	Romania
6.3%	2.5%	0.0%	99%	1.1%	150	Russia

Countries	Life expectancy At birth 2005	Maternal deaths Per 100,000 live births 2000	Under-five deaths Per 1,000 live births 2005	Cancer deaths	CVD deaths	Diabetes % of population with conditi 2003
				age-standardized mortality rate per 100,000 people 2002		
Rwanda	44	1,400	203	150	425	1.1%
Samoa	71	130	29	95	417	5.9%
São Tomé and Principe	63	–	118	133	396	2.8%
Saudi Arabia	72	23	26	109	405	9.4%
Senegal	56	690	136	146	426	2.3%
Serbia*	74	–	9	149	508	5.6%
Seychelles	–	–	13	131	336	12.3%
Sierra Leone	41	2,000	282	181	515	2.2%
Singapore	79	30	3	128	171	12.3%
Slovakia	74	3	9	170	371	8.7%
Slovenia	77	17	4	160	228	9.6%
Solomon Islands	63	130	29	90	409	2.1%
Somalia	47	1,100	225	143	580	2.3%
South Africa	46	230	68	154	410	3.4%
Spain	80	4	5	131	137	9.9%
Sri Lanka	74	92	14	118	314	2.1%
St. Kitts and Nevis	–	–	20	108	420	6.6%
St. Lucia	73	–	14	129	304	6.2%
St. Vincent and Grenadines	71	–	20	155	315	7.7%
Sudan	57	590	90	112	499	3.1%
Suriname	70	110	39	133	421	8.6%
Swaziland	30	370	160	162	364	3.0%
Sweden	80	2	4	116	176	7.3%
Switzerland	81	7	5	116	142	9.5%
Syria	74	160	15	60	410	6.2%
Tajikistan	64	100	71	90	753	3.7%
Tanzania	46	1,500	122	151	435	2.3%
Thailand	71	44	21	129	199	2.1%
Togo	55	570	139	147	427	2.1%
Tonga	73	–	24	85	363	12.4%
Trinidad and Tobago	70	160	19	121	379	7.9%
Tunisia	74	120	24	78	417	4.6%
Turkey	69	70	29	95	542	7.0%
Turkmenistan	63	31	104	99	844	4.0%
Tuvalu	–	–	38	129	541	8.6%
Uganda	49	880	136	146	422	1.5%
Ukraine	66	35	17	139	637	9.7%
United Arab Emirates	79	54	9	100	369	20.1%
United Kingdom	79	13	6	143	182	3.9%
United States	78	17	8	134	188	8.0%
Uruguay	76	27	15	170	208	6.8%
Uzbekistan	67	24	68	74	663	4.0%
Vanuatu	69	130	38	92	409	2.2%
Venezuela	73	96	21	107	241	5.2%
Vietnam	71	130	19	123	318	1.0%
Yemen	62	570	102	108	553	7.7%
Zambia	38	750	182	122	359	3.0%
Zimbabwe	37	1,100	86	122	347	2.6%

 * The data for Serbia and Montenegro predate their separation in 2006.

Deaths of under-fives Cause of death as % of all deaths			Measles % of infants receiving dose of vaccine 2005	HIV/AIDS % of people aged 15–49 with HIV 2005	Tuberculosis Number of cases per 100,000 people 2005	Countries
umonia 2000	diarrhoea 2000	malaria 2000				
23.2%	18.5%	4.6%	89%	3.1%	673	Rwanda
10.2%	9.7%	0.1%	57%	–	27	Samoa
21.2%	16.0%	0.6%	88%	–	258	São Tomé and Principe
6.6%	6.2%	0.2%	96%	–	58	Saudi Arabia
20.7%	17.1%	27.6%	74%	0.9%	466	Senegal
9.1%	6.0%	0.0%	96%	0.2%	42	Serbia*
10.1%	0.0%	0.0%	99%	–	56	Seychelles
25.5%	19.7%	12.4%	67%	1.6%	905	Sierra Leone
9.0%	0.4%	0.0%	96%	0.3%	28	Singapore
9.4%	1.4%	0.0%	98%	<0.1	20	Slovakia
0.0%	0.0%	0.0%	94%	<0.1	15	Slovenia
9.5%	8.8%	0.1%	72%	–	201	Solomon Islands
23.9%	18.7%	4.5%	35%	0.9%	286	Somalia
0.9%	0.8%	0.0%	82%	18.8%	511	South Africa
1.3%	0.1%	0.0%	97%	0.6%	22	Spain
8.5%	13.5%	0.4%	99%	<0.1	80	Sri Lanka
0.0%	14.4%	0.0%	99%	–	17	St. Kitts and Nevis
1.3%	1.3%	0.0%	94%	–	22	St. Lucia
10.5%	0.5%	0.0%	97%	–	42	St. Vincent and Grenadines
15.5%	12.9%	21.2%	60%	1.6%	400	Sudan
11.5%	13.1%	2.4%	91%	1.9%	99	Suriname
11.8%	9.6%	0.2%	60%	33.4%	1,211	Swaziland
0.8%	0.0%	0.0%	94%	0.2%	5	Sweden
0.7%	0.2%	0.0%	82%	0.4%	6	Switzerland
9.9%	9.6%	0.2%	98%	–	46	Syria
19.9%	16.4%	0.8%	84%	0.1%	297	Tajikistan
21.1%	16.8%	22.7%	91%	6.5%	496	Tanzania
11.5%	16.2%	0.3%	96%	1.4%	204	Thailand
17.1%	13.8%	25.3%	70%	3.2%	753	Togo
7.3%	10.0%	1.3%	99%	–	32	Tonga
2.0%	1.3%	0.0%	93%	2.6%	13	Trinidad and Tobago
7.6%	7.0%	0.2%	96%	0.1%	28	Tunisia
14.0%	12.2%	0.5%	91%	–	44	Turkey
18.8%	15.6%	0.9%	99%	<0.1	90	Turkmenistan
13.5%	13.2%	0.0%	62%	–	495	Tuvalu
21.1%	17.2%	23.1%	86%	6.7%	559	Uganda
6.3%	1.2%	0.0%	96%	1.4%	120	Ukraine
4.7%	6.3%	0.0%	92%	–	24	United Arab Emirates
2.2%	0.9%	0.0%	82%	0.2%	11	United Kingdom
1.3%	0.1%	0.0%	93%	0.6%	3	United States
5.4%	2.3%	0.0%	95%	0.5%	33	Uruguay
16.8%	14.8%	0.8%	99%	0.2%	139	Uzbekistan
13.0%	11.5%	0.6%	70%	–	84	Vanuatu
5.9%	9.9%	0.0%	76%	0.7%	52	Venezuela
11.5%	10.4%	0.4%	95%	0.5%	235	Vietnam
19.8%	16.1%	7.5%	76%	–	136	Yemen
21.8%	17.5%	19.4%	84%	17.0%	618	Zambia
14.7%	12.1%	0.2%	85%	20.1%	631	Zimbabwe

Countries	Population		Gross National Income	Inequality ratio	Education Net primary enrolment 2004		Healthcare spending	Healthcare staff Per 10,000 people 2004 or latest available data		Wa % w acce impr sou
	thousands 2005	% aged 60 or over	US$ per capita 2005	Income of richest 20% to poorest 20% 2005	boys	girls	% of GDP	nurses	doctors	20
Afghanistan	29,863	4%	250	–	–	–	–	2	2	
Albania	3,130	12%	2,580	4.1	96	95	2.7%	36	13	96
Algeria	32,854	7%	2,730	6.1	98	95	3.3%	20	11	85
Angola	15,941	4%	1,350	–	–	–	2.4%	13	1	53
Antigua and Barbuda	81	–	10,920	–	–	–	3.2%	33	2	91
Argentina	38,747	14%	4,470	17.6	99	98	4.3%	8	30	96
Armenia	3,016	14%	1,470	5.0	92	95	1.2%	44	36	92
Australia	20,155	18%	32,220	7.0	96	96	6.4%	91	25	100
Austria	8,189	23%	36,980	4.4	–	–	5.1%	94	34	100
Azerbaijan	8,411	9%	1,240	2.6	85	83	0.9%	71	36	77
Bahamas	323	10%	14,920	–	83	85	3.0%	45	11	97
Bahrain	727	5%	10,840	–	96	97	2.8%	40	11	
Bangladesh	141,822	6%	470	4.6	92	95	1.1%	1	3	74
Barbados	270	14%	9,270	–	98	97	4.8%	37	12	100
Belarus	9,755	18%	2,760	4.5	91	88	3.9%	116	46	100
Belgium	10,419	23%	35,700	4.9	99	99	6.3%	58	45	
Belize	270	6%	3,500	–	95	96	2.2%	13	11	91
Benin	8,439	4%	510	6.0	93	72	1.9%	7	<1	67
Bhutan	2,163	7%	870	–	–	–	2.6%	1	1	62
Bolivia	9,182	7%	1,010	42.3	95	96	4.3%	22	12	85
Bosnia and Herzegovina	3,907	20%	2,440	3.8	–	–	4.8%	41	13	97
Botswana	1,765	6%	5,180	31.5	81	83	3.3%	27	4	95
Brazil	186,405	9%	3,460	23.7	–	–	3.4%	38	12	90
Brunei	374	5%	24,100	–	–	–	2.8%	27	10	
Bulgaria	7,726	23%	3,450	4.4	96	95	4.1%	38	36	99
Burkina Faso	13,228	4%	400	6.9	46	35	2.6%	3	1	61
Burma	50,519	8%	220	–	89	91	0.5%	2	4	78
Burundi	7,548	4%	100	9.5	60	54	0.7%	2	<1	79
Cambodia	14,071	6%	380	6.9	100	96	2.1%	6	2	41
Cameroon	16,322	6%	1,010	9.1	–	–	1.2%	16	2	66
Canada	32,268	19%	32,600	5.5	99	100	6.9%	100	21	100
Cape Verde	507	5%	1,870	–	92	91	3.4%	9	5	80
Central African Republic	4,038	6%	350	32.7	–	–	1.5%	2	1	75
Chad	9,749	5%	400	–	68	46	2.6%	2	<1	42
Chile	16,295	20%	5,870	18.7	–	–	3.0%	6	11	95
China	1,315,844	12%	1,740	10.7	99	99	2.0%	11	11	77
Colombia	45,600	11%	2,290	25.3	83	84	6.4%	6	14	93
Comoros	798	8%	640	–	60	50	1.5%	6	2	86
Congo	3,999	4%	950	–	–	–	1.3%	8	2	58
Congo, Dem. Rep.	57,549	5%	120	–	–	–	0.7%	5	1	46
Cook Islands	18	4%	–	–	78	77	–	27	8	
Costa Rica	4,327	9%	4,590	14.2	–	–	5.8%	9	13	97
Côte d'Ivoire	18,154	5%	840	9.7	62	50	1.0%	5	1	84
Croatia	4,551	23%	8,060	4.8	88	87	6.5%	51	24	100
Cuba	11,269	16%	1,170	–	97	95	6.3%	74	59	91
Cyprus	835	17%	17,580	–	96	96	3.1%	38	23	100
Czech Republic	10,220	21%	10,710	3.5	–	–	6.8%	97	35	100
Denmark	5,431	22%	47,390	4.3	100	100	7.5%	104	29	100

DETERMINANTS AND CHALLENGES

Sanitation % with access to improved facilities 2004	Nutrition Average kCal consumed per person per day 2001–03	Underweight under-fives As % of total *latest available data 1996–2004*	Overweight under-fives As % of total *latest available data 1997-2006*	Tobacco % of adults who smoke cigarettes *2005 or latest available data*		Alcohol Average adult consumption of pure alcohol (litres) *2003*	Countries
				men	women		
–	–	–	–	–	–	0.0	Afghanistan
91%	2,860	–	30%	60.0%	18.0%	2.0	Albania
92%	3,040	10%	15%	32.3%	0.4%	0.2	Algeria
31%	2,070	31%	5%	–	–	3.9	Angola
95%	2,320	10%	–	–	–	5.7	Antigua and Barbuda
91%	2,980	5%	10%	32.3%	24.9%	8.4	Argentina
83%	2,260	–	12%	61.8%	2.4%	1.5	Armenia
100%	3,120	–	–	25.4%	19.5%	9.0	Australia
100%	3,740	–	–	33.9%	24.2%	11.1	Austria
54%	2,620	–	6%	30.2%	0.6%	4.5	Azerbaijan
100%	2,710	–	–	19.3%	3.8%	10.4	Bahamas
–	–	9%	–	15.0%	3.1%	7.0	Bahrain
39%	2,200	48%	1%	54.8%	26.7%	0.0	Bangladesh
100%	3,110	6%	–	20.1%	0.8%	–	Barbados
84%	2,960	–	–	53.2%	7.1%	5.5	Belarus
–	3,640	–	–	30.0%	25.0%	10.6	Belgium
47%	2,840	6%	–	–	–	6.3	Belize
33%	2,530	23%	3%	–	–	1.3	Benin
70%	–	19%	4%	–	–	0.2	Bhutan
46%	2,220	8%	9%	37.6%	19.4%	3.2	Bolivia
95%	2,710	–	16%	49.2%	29.7%	9.1	Bosnia and Herzegovina
42%	2,180	13%	10%	–	–	4.3	Botswana
75%	3,060	6%	–	21.8%	14.0%	5.8	Brazil
–	2,850	–	–	–	–	0.1	Brunei
99%	2,850	–	14%	43.8%	23.0%	5.9	Bulgaria
13%	2,460	38%	5%	–	–	5.0	Burkina Faso
77%	2,900	32%	2%	36.4%	12.2%	0.3	Burma
36%	1,640	45%	1%	15.6%	11.4%	9.1	Burundi
17%	2,060	45%	4%	66.7%	10.0%	1.5	Cambodia
51%	2,270	18%	9%	–	–	3.8	Cameroon
100%	3,590	–	–	19.0%	14.0%	7.8	Canada
43%	3,220	14%	–	–	–	4.8	Cape Verde
27%	1,940	24%	11%	–	–	1.5	Central African Republic
9%	2,160	28%	4%	24.1%	–	0.3	Chad
91%	2,860	1%	12%	48.3%	36.8%	6.6	Chile
44%	2,940	8%	6%	67.0%	1.9%	5.2	China
86%	2,580	7%	4%	26.8%	11.3%	5.7	Colombia
33%	1,750	25%	22%	–	–	0.3	Comoros
27%	2,150	14%	9%	–	–	2.6	Congo
30%	1,610	31%	7%	–	–	1.9	Congo, Dem. Rep.
–	–	–	–	34.4%	71.1%	3.7	Cook Islands
92%	2,850	5%	–	29.0%	9.7%	5.7	Costa Rica
37%	2,630	17%	5%	42.3%	1.8%	1.8	Côte d'Ivoire
100%	2,770	–	–	34.1%	26.6%	12.3	Croatia
98%	3,190	4%	–	48.1%	26.2%	2.3	Cuba
100%	3,240	–	–	38.5%	7.6%	11.5	Cyprus
98%	3,240	–	4%	31.1%	20.1%	13.0	Czech Republic
–	3,450	–	–	31.0%	25.0%	11.7	Denmark

111

Countries	Population		Gross National Income US$ per capita 2005	Inequality ratio Income of richest 20% to poorest 20% 2005	Education Net primary enrolment 2004		Healthcare spending % of GDP	Healthcare staff Per 10,000 people 2004 or latest available data		Wat* % w acces impro sou 200
	thousands 2005	% aged 60 or over			boys	girls		nurses	doctors	
Djibouti	793	5%	1,020	–	36	29	3.8%	3	2	73*
Dominica	79	–	3,790	–	87	88	4.5%	42	5	97*
Dominican Republic	8,895	7%	2,370	14.4	85	87	2.3%	18	19	95
East Timor	947	5%	750	–	–	–	7.3%	18	1	58
Ecuador	13,228	9%	2,630	17.3	97	98	2.0%	16	15	94
Egypt	74,033	7%	1,250	5.1	97	94	2.5%	20	5	98*
El Salvador	6,881	8%	2,450	20.9	92	92	3.7%	8	12	84
Equatorial Guinea	504	6%	–	–	92	78	1.0%	4	3	43*
Eritrea	4,401	4%	220	–	50	42	2.0%	6	1	60*
Estonia	1,330	22%	9,100	6.4	94	94	4.1%	85	45	100*
Ethiopia	77,431	5%	160	4.3	58	55	3.4%	2	<1	22*
Fiji	848	7%	3,280	–	97	96	2.3%	20	3	47*
Finland	5,249	23%	37,460	3.8	99	99	5.7%	143	32	100*
France	60,496	22%	34,810	5.6	99	99	7.7%	72	34	100*
Gabon	1,384	6%	5,010	–	77	77	2.9%	46	3	88*
Gambia	1,517	6%	290	11.2	73	77	3.2%	11	1	82*
Georgia	4,474	18%	1,350	8.3	93	92	1.0%	35	41	82*
Germany	82,689	25%	34,580	4.3	–	–	8.7%	97	34	100*
Ghana	22,113	6%	450	8.4	65	65	1.4%	7	2	75*
Greece	11,120	23%	19,670	6.2	100	99	5.1%	39	44	
Grenada	103	–	3,920	–	84	84	4.9%	37	5	95*
Guatemala	12,599	6%	2,400	20.3	95	91	2.1%	41	9	95*
Guinea	9,402	6%	370	7.3	69	58	0.9%	5	1	50*
Guinea-Bissau	1,586	5%	180	10.3	53	37	2.6%	6	1	59*
Guyana	751	8%	1,010	–	–	–	4.0%	23	5	83*
Haiti	8,528	6%	450	26.6	–	–	2.9%	1	3	54*
Honduras	7,205	6%	1,190	17.2	90	92	4.0%	13	6	87*
Hungary	10,098	21%	10,030	3.8	90	88	6.1%	89	33	99*
Iceland	295	16%	46,320	–	100	98	8.8%	136	36	100*
India	1,103,371	8%	720	4.9	92	87	1.2%	8	6	86*
Indonesia	222,781	9%	1,280	5.2	95	93	1.1%	6	1	77*
Iran	69,515	7%	2,770	9.7	89	88	3.1%	12	9	94*
Iraq	28,807	5%	2,170	–	94	81	–	13	7	
Ireland	4,148	16%	40,150	5.6	96	96	5.8%	152	28	
Israel	6,725	14%	18,620	7.9	97	98	6.1%	63	38	100*
Italy	58,093	26%	30,010	6.5	99	99	6.3%	54	42	
Jamaica	2,651	10%	3,400	6.9	90	91	2.7%	17	9	93*
Japan	128,085	28%	38,980	3.4	100	100	6.4%	78	20	100*
Jordan	5,703	5%	2,500	6.9	90	92	4.2%	29	20	97*
Kazakhstan	14,825	11%	2,930	5.6	93	92	2.0%	60	35	86*
Kenya	34,256	4%	530	8.2	76	77	1.7%	12	1	61*
Kiribati	99	–	1,390	–	96	98	–	24	3	
Korea, North	22,488	12%	–	4.7	–	–	–	39	33	
Korea, South	47,817	15%	15,830	–	100	99	2.8%	18	16	92*
Kuwait	2,687	3%	16,340	–	85	87	2.7%	39	15	
Kyrgyzstan	5,264	8%	440	4.4	90	90	2.2%	61	25	77*
Laos	5,924	5%	440	5.4	87	82	1.2%	–	–	51*
Latvia	2,307	23%	6,760	6.8	–	–	3.3%	53	30	99*

DETERMINANTS AND CHALLENGES

...itation with ...ess to ...roved ...ilities ...004	Nutrition Average kCal consumed per person per day 2001–03	Underweight under-fives As % of total latest available data 1996–2004	Overweight under-fives As % of total latest available data 1997-2006	Tobacco % of adults who smoke cigarettes 2005 or latest available data		Alcohol Average adult consumption of pure alcohol (litres) 2003	Countries
				men	women		
82%	–	18%	–	75.0%	10.0%	1.8	Djibouti
84%	2,770	5%	–	–	–	7.5	Dominica
78%	2,290	5%	9%	15.8%	10.9%	6.7	Dominican Republic
36%	–	46%	6%	–	1.1%	_	East Timor
89%	2,710	12%	5%	45.5%	17.4%	2.4	Ecuador
70%	3,350	9%	14%	45.4%	12.1%	0.2	Egypt
62%	2,560	10%	6%	38.0%	12.0%	3.7	El Salvador
53%	–	19%	14%	–	–	3.4	Equatorial Guinea
9%	1,520	40%	2%	–	–	0.6	Eritrea
97%	3,160	–	–	45.0%	17.9%	9.0	Estonia
13%	1,860	47%	5%	5.9%	0.3%	0.9	Ethiopia
72%	2,960	8%	–	26.0%	3.9%	1.7	Fiji
...00%	3,150	–	–	25.7%	19.3%	9.3	Finland
–	3,640	–	–	30.0%	21.2%	11.4	France
36%	2,670	12%	6%	–	–	8.0	Gabon
53%	2,280	17%	3%	38.5%	4.4%	2.6	Gambia
94%	2,520	–	18%	53.3%	6.3%	1.5	Georgia
...00%	3,490	–	–	37.3%	28.0%	12.0	Germany
18%	2,650	22%	5%	7.4%	0.7%	1.6	Ghana
–	3,680	–	–	46.8%	29.0%	9.0	Greece
96%	–	–	–	–	–	6.7	Grenada
86%	2,210	23%	6%	21.0%	2.0%	1.5	Guatemala
18%	2,420	21%	5%	58.9%	47.3%	0.2	Guinea
35%	2,070	25%	5%	–	–	2.2	Guinea-Bissau
70%	2,730	14%	6%	–	–	3.8	Guyana
30%	2,090	17%	3%	14.6%	6.1%	8.3	Haiti
69%	2,360	17%	6%	36.0%	11.0%	2.9	Honduras
95%	3,500	–	–	40.5%	27.8%	13.6	Hungary
...00%	3,240	–	–	25.4%	19.6%	7.0	Iceland
33%	2,440	47%	4%	46.6%	16.8%	0.3	India
55%	2,880	28%	5%	58.3%	2.9%	0.1	Indonesia
–	3,090	11%	7%	22.0%	2.1%	0.0	Iran
–	–	–	6%	40.0%	5.0%	0.2	Iraq
–	3,690	–	–	28.0%	26.0%	13.7	Ireland
–	3,680	–	–	31.9%	17.8%	2.5	Israel
–	3,670	–	–	31.3%	17.2%	8.0	Italy
80%	2,680	4%	8%	37.7%	11.6%	1.7	Jamaica
...00%	2,770	–	–	46.9%	14.5%	7.6	Japan
93%	2,680	4%	5%	50.5%	8.3%	0.3	Jordan
72%	2,710	–	5%	65.3%	9.3%	3.0	Kazakhstan
43%	2,150	20%	6%	21.3%	1.0%	1.5	Kenya
–	–	–	–	56.5%	32.3%	0.5	Kiribati
–	2,160	–	1%	–	–	3.3	Korea, North
–	3,040	–	–	64.9%	4.4%	7.9	Korea, South
–	3,060	10%	9%	34.4%	1.9%	0.0	Kuwait
59%	3,050	–	9%	51.0%	4.5%	3.6	Kyrgyzstan
30%	2,320	40%	3%	58.7%	12.5%	6.9	Laos
78%	3,020	–	–	51.1%	19.2%	9.6	Latvia

113

| Countries | Population | | Gross National Income | Inequality ratio | Education | | Healthcare spending | Healthcare staff | | Wa |
| | thousands 2005 | % aged 60 or over | US$ per capita 2005 | Income of richest 20% to poorest 20% 2005 | Net primary enrolment 2004 | | % of GDP | Per 10,000 people 2004 or latest available data | | % w acce impr sou 20 |
					boys	girls		nurses	doctors	
Lebanon	3,577	10%	6,180	–	94	93	3.0%	12	33	100
Lesotho	1,795	8%	960	44.2	83	88	4.1%	6	1	79
Liberia	3,283	4%	130	–	74	58	–	2	<1	
Libya	5,853	7%	5,530	–	–	–	2.6%	36	13	
Lithuania	3,431	21%	7,050	6.3	90	89	5.0%	76	40	
Luxembourg	465	18%	65,630	–	91	91	6.2%	92	27	100
Macedonia	2,034	16%	2,830	7.5	92	92	6.0%	52	22	
Madagascar	18,606	5%	290	11.0	89	89	1.7%	2	3	50
Malawi	12,884	5%	160	11.6	93	98	3.3%	6	<1	73
Malaysia	25,347	7%	4,960	12.4	93	93	2.2%	14	7	99
Maldives	329	5%	2,390	–	89	90	5.5%	27	9	83
Mali	13,518	4%	380	12.2	50	43	2.8%	5	1	50
Malta	402	20%	13,590	–	94	94	7.4%	58	32	100
Marshall Islands	62	–	2,930	–	90	89	–	30	5	
Mauritania	3,069	5%	560	7.4	75	74	3.2%	6	1	53
Mauritius	1,245	10%	5,260	–	94	95	2.2%	36	11	100
Mexico	107,029	8%	7,310	12.8	98	98	2.9%	9	20	97
Micronesia, Fed. Sts.	110	5%	2,300	–	–	–	–	38	6	
Moldova	4,206	14%	880	5.3	86	86	3.9%	61	26	92
Mongolia	2,646	6%	690	9.1	84	84	4.3%	32	26	62
Montenegro*	10,503	19%	3,280	–	96	96	–	46	21	
Morocco	31,478	7%	1,730	7.2	89	83	1.7%	7	5	81
Mozambique	19,792	5%	310	7.2	75	67	2.9%	2	<1	43
Namibia	2,031	6%	2,990	56.1	71	76	4.5%	31	3	87
Nauru	14	–	–	–	–	–	–	–	–	
Nepal	27,133	6%	270	9.1	83	73	1.5%	2	2	90
Netherlands	16,299	20%	36,620	5.1	99	98	6.1%	137	32	100
New Zealand	4,028	17%	25,960	6.8	99	99	6.3%	82	24	
Nicaragua	5,487	5%	910	8.8	89	87	3.7%	11	4	79
Niger	13,957	3%	240	20.7	46	32	2.5%	2	<1	46
Nigeria	131,530	5%	560	9.7	64	57	1.3%	10	3	48
Niue	1	–	–	–	99	98	–	148	31	
Norway	4,620	21%	59,590	3.9	99	99	8.6%	–	–	100
Oman	2,567	4%	7,830	–	77	79	2.7%	35	13	
Pakistan	157,935	6%	690	4.3	76	56	0.7%	3	7	91
Palau	20	–	7,630	–	98	94	–	14	11	
Palestine Authority	3,702	4%	1,110	–	86	86	–	–	–	92
Panama	3,232	9%	4,630	23.9	98	98	5.0%	28	15	90
Papua New Guinea	5,887	4%	660	12.6	–	–	3.0%	5	1	39
Paraguay	6,158	6%	1,280	27.8	–	–	2.3%	17	11	86
Peru	27,968	8%	2,610	18.6	97	97	2.1%	7	12	83
Philippines	83,054	6%	1,300	9.7	93	95	1.4%	17	6	85
Poland	38,530	17%	7,110	5.6	97	98	4.5%	49	25	
Portugal	10,495	23%	16,170	8.0	99	99	6.7%	44	34	
Puerto Rico	–	18%	–	–	–	–	–	–	–	
Qatar	813	3%	12,000	–	95	94	2.0%	49	22	100
Romania	21,711	20%	3,830	4.9	92	92	3.8%	39	19	57
Russia	143,202	17%	4,460	7.6	91	92	3.3%	81	43	97

   * The data for Serbia and Montenegro predate their separation in 2006.

...itation with ...ess to ...roved ...ilities ...004	Nutrition Average kCal consumed per person per day 2001–03	Underweight under-fives As % of total latest available data 1996–2004	Overweight under-fives As % of total latest available data 1997-2006	Tobacco % of adults who smoke cigarettes 2005 or latest available data men	Tobacco women	Alcohol Average adult consumption of pure alcohol (litres) 2003	Countries
98%	3,170	3%	–	42.3%	30.6%	3.2	Lebanon
37%	2,630	18%	21%	38.5%	1.0%	1.8	Lesotho
–	1,940	–	5%	–	–	3.8	Liberia
97%	3,330	5%	–	–	–	0.0	Libya
–	3,370	–	–	43.7%	12.8%	9.9	Lithuania
–	3,710	–	–	39.0%	26.0%	15.6	Luxembourg
–	2,800	–	8%	40.0%	32.0%	5.7	Macedonia
34%	2,040	42%	6%	–	–	1.6	Madagascar
61%	2,140	22%	10%	20.5%	4.8%	1.4	Malawi
94%	2,870	11%	6%	43.0%	1.6%	1.1	Malaysia
59%	–	30%	4%	37.4%	15.6%	–	Maldives
46%	2,230	33%	3%	–	–	0.5	Mali
–	3,530	–	–	29.9%	17.6%	6.0	Malta
–	–	–	–	–	–	–	Marshall Islands
34%	2,780	32%	4%	–	–	0.0	Mauritania
94%	2,960	15%	–	32.1%	1.0%	3.0	Mauritius
79%	3,180	8%	8%	12.9%	4.7%	4.6	Mexico
–	–	–	–	42.0%	0.0%	1.2	Micronesia, Fed. Sts.
68%	2,730	–	9%	33.6%	1.8%	13.2	Moldova
59%	2,250	13%	6%	52.4%	7.5%	2.8	Mongolia
–	2,670	–	–	48.0%	33.6%	–	*Montenegro
73%	3,070	9%	13%	28.5%	0.1%	0.5	Morocco
32%	2,070	24%	6%	–	–	0.5	Mozambique
25%	2,260	24%	3%	22.8%	9.6%	6.0	Namibia
–	–	–	–	49.8%	59.0%	0.9	Nauru
35%	2,450	48%	1%	48.5%	24.0%	0.2	Nepal
00%	3,440	–	–	35.8%	28.4%	9.7	Netherlands
–	3,200	–	–	23.7%	22.2%	9.7	New Zealand
47%	2,290	10%	7%	–	5.3%	2.5	Nicaragua
13%	2,160	40%	2%	–	–	0.1	Niger
44%	2,700	29%	6%	15.4%	0.5%	10.6	Nigeria
–	–	–	–	37.5%	14.5%	9.5	Niue
–	3,480	–	–	27.2%	24.8%	5.5	Norway
–	–	24%	2%	15.5%	1.5%	0.3	Oman
59%	2,340	38%	5%	28.5%	3.4%	0.0	Pakistan
–	–	–	–	14.0%	4.0%	–	Palau
73%	2,240	4%	–	40.7%	3.2%	–	Palestine Authority
73%	2,260	7%	6%	19.7%	6.1%	6.0	Panama
44%	–	35%	–	46.0%	28.0%	1.6	Papua New Guinea
80%	2,530	5%	–	23.4%	6.8%	3.7	Paraguay
63%	2,570	7%	12%	52.5%	17.8%	3.8	Peru
72%	2,450	28%	2%	40.5%	7.6%	3.5	Philippines
–	3,370	–	–	40.0%	25.0%	8.1	Poland
–	3,750	–	–	32.8%	9.5%	11.5	Portugal
–	–	–	–	16.8%	9.9%	–	Puerto Rico
00%	–	6%	–	37.0%	0.5%	4.4	Qatar
–	3,520	–	8%	32.3%	10.1%	9.7	Romania
87%	3,080	–	–	60.4%	15.5%	10.3	Russia

Countries	Population thousands 2005	Population % aged 60 or over	Gross National Income US$ per capita 2005	Inequality ratio Income of richest 20% to poorest 20% 2005	Education Net primary enrolment 2004 boys	Education girls	Healthcare spending % of GDP	Healthcare staff Per 10,000 people 2004 or latest available data nurses	doctors	Wa % w acce impr sou 20
Rwanda	9,038	4%	230	4.0	72	75	1.6%	4	1	74
Samoa	185	7%	2,090	–	90	91	4.3%	20	7	88
São Tomé and Principe	157	5%	390	–	98	98	7.2%	16	5	79
Saudi Arabia	24,573	5%	11,770	–	62	57	3.0%	30	14	
Senegal	11,658	5%	710	7.5	68	64	2.1%	3	1	76
Serbia*	10,503	19%	3,280	–	96	96	–	46	21	
Seychelles	81	–	8,290	–	96	97	4.3%	79	15	88
Sierra Leone	5,525	6%	220	57.6	–	–	2.0%	2	<1	57
Singapore	4,326	14%	27,490	9.7	–	–	1.6%	42	14	100
Slovakia	5,401	17%	7,950	4.0	–	–	5.2%	68	32	100
Slovenia	1,967	21%	17,350	3.9	98	98	6.7%	72	23	
Solomon Islands	478	4%	590	–	80	79	4.5%	8	1	70
Somalia	8,228	4%	130	–	–	–	–	2	<1	
South Africa	47,432	7%	4,960	17.9	88	89	3.2%	41	8	88
Spain	43,064	22%	25,360	6.0	100	99	5.5%	77	33	100
Sri Lanka	20,743	11%	1,160	5.1	99	98	1.6%	12	6	79
St. Kitts and Nevis	43	–	8,210	–	91	98	3.4%	50	12	100
St. Lucia	161	10%	4,800	–	99	96	3.4%	23	52	98
St. Vincent and Grenadines	119	9%	3,590	–	95	92	4.1%	24	9	
Sudan	36,233	6%	640	–	47	39	1.9%	5	2	70
Suriname	449	9%	2,540	–	90	96	3.6%	16	5	92
Swaziland	1,032	6%	2,280	23.8	76	77	3.3%	42	2	62
Sweden	9,041	24%	41,060	4.0	99	98	8.0%	102	33	100
Switzerland	7,252	23%	54,930	5.5	94	94	6.7%	108	36	100
Syria	19,043	5%	1,380	–	97	92	2.5%	19	14	93
Tajikistan	6,507	5%	330	5.2	99	94	0.9%	46	20	59
Tanzania	38,329	5%	340	5.8	92	91	2.4%	3	<1	62
Thailand	64,233	11%	2,750	7.7	–	–	2.0%	28	4	99
Togo	6,145	5%	350	–	85	72	1.4%	3	<1	52
Tonga	102	9%	2,190	–	92	89	5.5%	32	3	100
Trinidad and Tobago	1,305	11%	10,440	8.3	92	92	1.5%	29	8	91
Tunisia	10,102	9%	2,890	7.9	97	98	2.5%	26	13	93
Turkey	73,193	8%	4,710	9.3	92	87	5.4%	17	14	96
Turkmenistan	4,833	6%	1,340	7.7	–	–	2.6%	90	42	72
Tuvalu	10	–	–	–	–	–	–	26	6	
Uganda	28,816	4%	280	8.4	–	–	2.2%	6	1	60
Ukraine	46,481	21%	1,520	4.1	82	82	3.8%	76	30	96
United Arab Emirates	4,496	2%	18,060	–	72	70	2.5%	42	20	100
United Kingdom	59,668	22%	37,600	7.2	99	99	6.9%	121	23	100
United States	298,213	17%	43,740	8.4	94	90	6.8%	94	26	100
Uruguay	3,463	18%	4,360	10.2	–	–	2.7%	9	37	100
Uzbekistan	26,593	6%	510	4.0	–	–	2.4%	98	27	82
Vanuatu	211	5%	1,600	–	95	93	2.9%	24	1	60
Venezuela	26,749	8%	4,810	10.6	92	92	2.0%	7	19	83
Vietnam	84,238	7%	620	6.0	97	91	1.5%	6	5	85
Yemen	20,975	4%	600	5.6	87	63	2.2%	6	3	67
Zambia	11,668	5%	490	8.0	80	80	2.8%	16	1	58
Zimbabwe	13,010	6%	340	12.0	81	82	2.8%	7	2	81

   * The data for Serbia and Montenegro predate their separation in 2006.

tation with ess to roved ilities 004	Nutrition Average kCal consumed per person per day 2001–03	Underweight under-fives As % of total latest available data 1996–2004	Overweight under-fives As % of total latest available data 1997-2006	Tobacco % of adults who smoke cigarettes 2005 or latest available data		Alcohol Average adult consumption of pure alcohol (litres) 2003	Countries
				men	women		
42%	2,070	27%	7%	7.0%	4.0%	6.9	Rwanda
00%	2,910	–	7%	60.0%	24.0%	–	Samoa
25%	2,440	13%	9%	–	–	7.0	São Tomé and Principe
–	2,820	14%	–	14.4%	4.9%	0.0	Saudi Arabia
57%	2,310	23%	2%	–	–	0.5	Senegal
–	2,670	–	–	48.0%	33.6%	–	*Serbia
–	2,460	6%	–	37.0%	6.9%	3.4	Seychelles
39%	1,930	27%	5%	40.8%	7.4%	6.4	Sierra Leone
00%	–	14%	3%	24.2%	3.5%	2.2	Singapore
99%	2,830	–	–	41.1%	14.7%	10.4	Slovakia
–	2,970	–	–	28.0%	20.1%	6.7	Slovenia
31%	2,250	21%	–	–	23.0%	1.0	Solomon Islands
–	–	–	–	–	–	0.0	Somalia
65%	2,940	12%	9%	23.2%	7.7%	6.7	South Africa
00%	3,410	–	–	39.2%	24.6%	11.7	Spain
91%	2,390	29%	1%	23.2%	1.7%	0.3	Sri Lanka
95%	2,700	–	–	–	–	6.7	St. Kitts and Nevis
89%	2,960	14%	–	37.3%	5.6%	11.5	St. Lucia
–	2,580	–	–	17.4%	1.9%	7.0	St. Vincent and Grenadines
34%	2,260	17%	5%	23.5%	1.5%	0.3	Sudan
94%	2,660	13%	3%	–	–	–	Suriname
48%	2,360	10%	15%	10.5%	2.9%	4.6	Swaziland
00%	3,160	–	–	16.7%	18.3%	6.0	Sweden
00%	3,500	–	–	26.5%	23.1%	10.8	Switzerland
90%	3,060	7%	–	–	–	0.5	Syria
51%	1,840	–	–	–	–	0.4	Tajikistan
47%	1,960	22%	5%	23.0%	1.3%	5.5	Tanzania
99%	2,410	19%	10%	48.5%	2.9%	5.6	Thailand
35%	2,320	25%	3%	–	–	1.2	Togo
96%	–	–	–	52.9%	10.5%	0.8	Tonga
00%	2,770	7%	5%	42.4%	4.2%	4.2	Trinidad and Tobago
85%	3,250	4%	7%	49.5%	2.4%	1.2	Tunisia
88%	3,340	4%	4%	49.4%	17.6%	1.4	Turkey
62%	2,750	–	–	27.0%	1.0%	1.2	Turkmenistan
–	–	–	–	51.0%	31.0%	1.4	Tuvalu
43%	2,380	23%	5%	25.2%	3.3%	17.6	Uganda
96%	3,030	–	27%	52.5%	11.1%	6.1	Ukraine
98%	3,220	14%	–	17.3%	1.3%	0.0	United Arab Emirates
–	3,440	–	–	27.0%	25.0%	11.8	United Kingdom
00%	3,770	–	7%	19.8%	15.9%	8.6	United States
00%	2,850	5%	9%	34.6%	23.8%	7.7	Uruguay
67%	2,270	–	–	24.1%	0.9%	1.5	Uzbekistan
50%	2,590	20%	–	49.1%	5.0%	0.8	Vanuatu
68%	2,350	4%	6%	35.9%	21.4%	6.7	Venezuela
61%	2,580	28%	3%	35.3%	1.7%	0.9	Vietnam
43%	2,020	46%	4%	77.0%	29.0%	0.0	Yemen
55%	1,930	23%	6%	16.0%	1.0%	2.4	Zambia
53%	2,010	13%	11%	20.0%	2.2%	4.4	Zimbabwe

SOURCES

Foreword
"....if physicians were to read" William F Miser. Critical Appraisal of the Literature. Journal of the American Board of Family Practice. 12 (4):315-333, 1999.

Introduction
Commission on Social Determinants of Health. http://www.who.int/social_determinants/en/

Dahlgren G, Whitehead M. European strategies for tackling social inequities in health: levelling up Part 2. Copenhagen: WHO Regional Office for Europe; 2006.

Donaldson L, Banatvala N. Health is global: proposals for a UK government-wide strategy. Lancet 2007;369:857-61

Farmer P. Infections and inequalities. The modern plague. Berkeley and Los Angeles: University of California Press; 1999.

Farmer P. Pathologies of power. Health, human rights and the new war on the poor. Berkeley and Los Angeles: University of California Press; 2003

Garrett L. Betrayal of Trust. The collapse of global public health. Oxford: Oxford University Press; 2001.

Global Health Watch 2005-2006. An alternative world health report. London: Zed Books; London 2005 (in association with People's Health Movement, Bangalore, Medact, London, Global Equity Gauge Alliance, Durban.)

Hunt P. The human right to the highest attainable standard of health: new opportunities and challenges. Transactions of the Royal Society of Tropical Medicine and Hygiene (2006);100:603-607

Institute of Medicine. The future of public health. Washington DC: National Academy Press; 1988.

Kawachi I, Wamala S (eds). Globalization and health. Oxford: Oxford University Press; 2007

Kickbusch I. The end of public health as we know it: constructing global health in the 21st century. Hugh R Leavell Lecture at the 10th International Congress on Public Health of the World Federation of Public Health Associations. http://www.ilonakickbusch.com/public-health/publichealthinteh21st.pdf

Lewis S. Race against time. Toronto: House of Anansi Press Inc; 2006.

Marmot M. Health in an unequal world. Lancet 2006;368:2081-94.

McKeown T. The origins of human disease. Oxford: Basil Blackwell;1988.

Organisation for Economic Co-operation and Development (OECD). International Development Statistics online. http://www.oecd.org/dataoecd/50/17/5037721.htm

Sen A. Development as freedom. Oxford: Oxford University Press; 1999.

UN Millennium Development Goals. http://www.un.org/millenniumgoals/

Wanless D. Securing our future health: Taking a long-term view. HM Treasury, London 2002.

Wilkinson R, Marmot M (eds). Social determinants of health (second edition). Oxford: Oxford University Press; 2005.

World Health Organization. http://www.who.int/en/

14–15 Part 1 A Picture of Health
Life Expectancy and Population
Department of Economic and Social Affairs: Population Division. World population prospects: The 2006 revision. Population database http://esa.un.org/unpp

16–17 LIFE EXPECTANCY
Fisher K & McKee M. Health and healthcare in transitional Europe. BMJ 2005;331:169-70.

Franco A, Alvarez-Dardet C, Ruiz MT. Effect of democracy on health: ecological study. BMJ 2004;329:1421-4.

Mathers CD, Ma Fat D, Inoue M, Rao C, Lopez AD. Counting the dead and what they died from: an assessment of the global status of cause of death data. Bulletin World Health Organization 2005;83:171-177.

McKee M & Nolte E. Lessons from health during the transition from communism. BMJ 2004;329:1428-9.

McMichael AJ, McKee M, Shkolnikov V, Valkonen V. Mortality trends and setbacks: global convergence or divergence? Lancet 2004;363:1155-9.

Life Expectancy
UNICEF. The state of the world's children 2007. New York: UNICEF; 2006. Table 1. Available at: http://www.unicef.org/sowc07/

Percentage of population aged under 15
Department of Economic and Social Affairs: Population Division. World population prospects: the 2006 revision. Table A.10

The Impact of AIDS
Population Division of the Department of Economic and Social Affairs of the United Nations Secretariat, World Population Prospects: The 2004 Revision and World Urbanization Prospects: The 2003 Revision.

18–19 MATERNAL HEALTH
Joint WHO/UNFPA/UNICEF/World Bank Statement. Reduction of Maternal Mortality. Geneva: WHO; 1999. www.safemotherhood.org

Maternal Mortality
Antenatal Care
UNICEF. The state of the world's children 2007. New York: UNICEF; 2006. Available at: http://www.unicef.org/sowc07/

Causes of Maternal Death
World Health Organization. World health report 2005. Geneva: WHO. 2005. Chapter 4 Available at: http://www.who.int/

20–21 CHILD HEALTH
UNICEF. The state of the world's children 2007. New York: UNICEF; 2006. Available at: http://www.unicef.org/sowc07/

The Partnership for Maternal, Newborn and Child Health. http://www.who.int/pmnch/en/

1970 mortality rates: UNDP. Human Development Report 2006. Beyond scarcity: Power, poverty and the global water crisis. New York: UNDP; 2006. Available at: http://hdr.undp.org/hdr2006/

Child Death Rate
World Health Organization Statistical Information System. http://www.who.int/whosis/

UNICEF. The state of the world's children 2007. New York: UNICEF; 2006. Table 1. Available at: http://www.unicef.org/sowc07/

Major Causes of Death
http://www.who.int/child-adolescent-health/overview/child_health/child_epidemiology.htm

22–23 Part 2 Determinants of Health
World Health Organization. World health report 2004. Changing history. Annex: Table 2. Available at: http://www.who.int/whr/2004/

Graphic based on: Dahlgren G, Whitehead M. European strategies for tackling social inequities in health: levelling up Part 2. Copenhagen: WHO Regional Office for Europe; 2006.

24–25 POVERTY AND INEQUALITY
Evans T, Whitehead M, Diderichsen F et al. editors. Challenging inequities in health. New York: Oxford University Press; 2001.

Marmot M. Health in an unequal world. Lancet 2006;368:2081-94.

Marmot M, Wilkinson RG, editors. Social determinants of health. Oxford: Oxford University Press; 1999.

United Nations. The Millennium Development Goals Report 2007. New York: United Nations. 2007. Available at: http://www.un.org/millenniumgoals/

Health and Poverty
World Health Organization Statistical Information System. http://www.who.int/whosis/

Human Poverty Index
Inequality ratio
UNDP. Human Development Report 2006. New York: UNDP; 2006. Available at: http://hdr.undp.org/hdr2006/

GNI below $350
World Bank. WDI database. Available at: http://web.worldbank.org/

Child Mortality and Poverty
Gwatkin D, Rutstein S, Johnson K, et al. Socioeconomic differences in health, nutrition and population. 2nd ed. Washington: World Bank; 2005. Available at: http://web.worldbank.org/

26–27 EDUCATION
UNAIDS. HIV/AIDS and education: a strategic approach. Geneva: UNAIDS; 2002.

UNESCO. Strong foundations: education for all global monitoring report 2007. Paris: UNESCO; 2006.

UNICEF. The state of the world's children 2007. New York: UNICEF; 2006.

UIS/UNICEF. Children out of school: measuring exclusion from primary education. Montreal/New York: UNESCO Institute for Statistics/UNICEF; 2005.

Female Education and Child Survival
Under-five mortality
UNICEF. 2007. op. cit. Table 5. Net primary school enrolment ratio for girls: the number in the official age-group for primary education as a percentage of the population in that age group.

Participation of girls
UNESCO. 2006. op. cit. Table 5.

Literacy Saves Lives
UNICEF. 2007. op. cit. Tables 1 & 5.

Fertility and Education
Department of Economic and Social Affairs: Population Division. World Population Prospects: The 2006 Revision: Population Database http://esa.un.org/unpp (accessed 8 Oct 2007).

UN Population Division Bangladesh http://www.unfpa-bangladesh.org:80/php/unfpa_pds_6.php

75% of children...
UIS/UNICEF. 2005. op.cit.

Two-thirds of illiterate adults are women...
UNESCO. 2006. op. cit.

Each year of a girl's education...
UNICEF. The state of the world's children 2004. New York: UNICEF; 2004.

28–29 FOOD AND NUTRITION
Joint WHO/FAO Expert consultation on diet, nutrition and the prevention of chronic diseases: Report of a joint WHO/FAO expert consultation, Geneva, 28 January-1 February 2002. WHO technical report series; 916. WHO, Geneva 2003. http://whqlibdoc.who.int/trs/WHO_TRS_916.pdf

World Health Organization. Globalization, diets and noncommunicable diseases. Geneva: WHO; 2002. http://whqlibdoc.who.int/publications/9241590416.pdf

United Nations Standing Committee on Nutrition. The fifth report on the world nutrition situation: Nutrition for improved development outcomes. SCN; 2004.

UNICEF. The state of the world's children 2007. New York: UNICEF; 2006.

World Health Organization. WHO Global strategy for food safety. WHO, Geneva 2002. Available at: http://www.who.int/

Calorific Intake
FAO. Statistical yearbook 2005-06, Table D.1.

Dental Caries
WHO Oral Health Country/Area Profile Programme http://www.whocollab.od.mah.se/expl/globalcar1.html

Increase in undernourished people
Proportion Undernourished
Food and Agriculture Organization of the United Nations. The state of food insecurity in the world 2006. Rome: FAO. 2006. Available at: http://www.fao.org/

30–31 WATER AND SANITATION
DfID. Addressing the water crisis: healthier and more productive lives for poor people. London: United Kingdom Department for International Development; 2001.

UNDP. Human Development Report 2006. Beyond scarcity: Power, poverty and the global water crisis.

New York: UNDP; 2006. Available at: http://hdr.undp.org/hdr2006/

UNICEF. The state of the world's children 2007. New York: UNICEF; 2006.

World Health Organization. The right to water. Geneva: WHO; 2003.

Access to Water
Access to Sanitation
UNDP. 2006. op. cit.

Diarrhoeal diseases
World Health Organization. Global burden of disease study 2004. Geneva: WHO; 2004.

Unequal Access
UNICEF. 2007. op. cit.

Nearly 6,000 children...
UNDP. 2006. op. cit.

88% of diarrhoeal disease...
United Nations Department of Economic and Social Affairs. The Millennium Development Goals Report. Statistical Annex 2006. New York: United Nations. 2006. Available at: http://mdgs.un.org/unsd/mdg/Default.aspx

32–33 HOUSING CONDITIONS
Rehfuess E, Mehta S, Pruss-Ustun A. Assessing household solid fuel use: Multiple implications for the Millennium Development Goals. Environmental Health Perspectives 2006;114:272-378 http://www.ehponline.org/docs/2006/8603/abstract.html

United Nations Human Settlements programme (UN-Habitat). The challenge of slums: global report on human settlements 2003. London: Earthscan; 2003.

UNICEF. The State of the World's Children 2006: Excluded and invisible. New York: UNICEF; 2006.

World Health Organization. Proceedings of the 2nd WHO International Housing and Health Symposium. Bonn: WHO Centre for Environment and Health; 2004.

World Health Organization. Estimated deaths & DALYs attributable to selected environmental risk factors 2002. http://www.who.int/quantifying_ehimpacts/countryprofilesebd.xls

Development of Slums
Slums
Urban Waste Management
UN-Habitat. The challenge of slums. op. cit.

Smoky Homes
Rehfuess E. op. cit.

34–35 WORKING CONDITIONS
Hagemann F, Diallo Y, Etienne A, Mehran F. Global child labour trends 2000 to 2004. Geneva: International Labour Office; 2006.

Lee S, McCann D, Messenger JC. Working time around the world: trends in working hours, laws and policies in a global comparative perspective. London and Geneva: Routledge and ILO; 2007.

Marmot M, Siegrist J, Theorell T, Feeney A. Health and the psychosocial environment at work. In Marmot & Wilkinson, editors. Social determinants of health. Oxford: Oxford University Press; 1999.

Benach J, Muntaner C, Santana V. http://www.who.int/social_determinants/resources/emconet_scoping_paper.pdf

Unemployment
United Nations Statistics Division. http://unstats.un.org/unsd/demographic/products/indwm/table%205f_2007.xls

Child Workers
Hagemann F. op. cit. 2006.

Youth Unemployment
International Labour Office. Global employment trends for youth. Geneva: ILO; 2004.

36–37 HEALTHCARE
Commission on Macroeconomics and Health. Macroeconomics and Health: Findings and Recommendations. WHO, 2003. http://www.who.int/macrohealth/events/en/cmh_rprt_overview_afro.pdf

Whitehead M, Dahlgren G, Evans T. Equity and health sector reforms: Can low income countries escape the medical poverty trap? Lancet 2001;358:833-36.

Public Expenditure
UNDP Human Development Report 2006. New York: UNDP; 2006. Available at: http://hdr.undp.org/hdr2006/

Inequality of Healthcare
Gwatkin D, Wagstaff A, Yazbeck AS (eds). Reaching the poor with health, nutrition and population services. Washington DC: World Bank; 2005. p7.

Hospital beds...
World Bank: World Development Indicators 2005. Washington DC: World Bank; 2005.

38–39 TOBACCO
Mackay J, Eriksen M, Shafey O. The tobacco atlas. Atlanta, Georgia: American Cancer Society; 2006.

World Health Organization. World health statistics 2007. Available at: http://www.who.int/whosis/

Smoking among Adults
Mackay, J. et al. The cancer atlas. Atlanta, Georgia: American Cancer Society; 2006.

Cancer Deaths Caused by Smoking
International Journal of Cancer, cited in Mackay, J. et al. The cancer atlas. 2006.

Tobacco Death Outlook
Peto R, Lopez AD. The future worldwide health effects of current smoking patterns. In: Koop EC, Pearson CE, Schwarz MR, editors. Critical issues in global health. New York: Jossey-Bass; 2001:154–61. Cited in Mackay J. et. al. The tobacco atlas. 2006. op. cit. p82.

Cost of Food and Tobacco
Economist Intelligence Unit. Worldwide cost of living. March 2003 http://eiu.enumerate.com/ Cited in Mackay J. et. al. The tobacco atlas. 2006. op. cit.
Union Bank of Switzerland (UBS). Prices and earnings. A comparison of purchasing power around the globe. 2003. Accessed Sept 2005. http://www.ubs.com/1/e/ubs_ch/wealth_mgmt_ch/research.html .
Cited in Mackay J. et. al. The tobacco atlas. 2006. op. cit.

40–41 ALCOHOL AND DRUGS
World Health Organization. World health statistics 2007. Highlights and Tables. Available at: http://www.who.int/whosis/

World Health Organization. Global Status Report on Alcohol 2004. Geneva: WHO; 2004. Available at: http://www.who.int

World Health Organization. Public health problems caused by harmful use of alcohol. Available at: http://www.who.int

Alcohol and Drug Use
World Health Organization Statistical Information System. http://www.who.int/whosis/

Opiates, Cocaine
Illegal Drug Use
United Nations Office on Drugs and Crime. World Drug Report 2007. Table 3.5.1. Available at: http://www.unodc.org/unodc/world_drug_report.html

42–43 Part 3 Health Problems

Major Causes of Death
Table 2, World Health Report 2004. Numbers rounded. Available at: http://www.who.int/

44–45 CANCER
Mackay J, Jemal A, Lee NC, Parkin DM. The cancer atlas. American Cancer Society, Atlanta; 2006.

World Health Organization. The World Health Organization's fight against cancer: Strategies that prevent, cure and care. Geneva: WHO; 2007.

Most Common Cancers
Global Differences
Ferlay J, Bray F, Pisani P, Parkin DM. IARC CancerBase No 5, version 2.0. Lyon: IARC Press, 2004.

Major Risk Factors
Mackay J op. cit. p24

Stewart BW and Kleihues P, editors. World cancer report. Lyon: IARC Press; 2003.

World Health Organization. Diet, nutrition and the prevention of chronic diseases. Geneva: WHO. Technical Report 2003; 916;95.S.

46–47 HEART DISEASE AND STROKE
Mackay J, Mensah GA. The atlas of heart disease and stroke. Geneva: WHO; 2004.

Strong K, Mathers C, Bonita R. Preventing stroke: saving lives around the world. Lancet Neurology 2007;6:182-7.

Cardiovascular Disease Deaths
World Health Organization Statistical Information System. http://www.who.int/whosis/

Strokes
World Health Organization. Global burden of disease estimates. Table 5. Age-standardized death rates per 100,000 (2002). http://www.who.int/healthinfo/statistics/bodgbddeathdalyestimates.xls

Major Risk Factors
World Health Organization. World Health Report 2002. Geneva: WHO; 2004. 57-61.

Coronary Heart Disease Death Rates
Mackay, J and Mensah, GA, op. cit.

48–49 DIABETES
International Diabetes Federation http://www.idf.org

Wild S, Roglic G, Green A, Sicree R, King H. Global prevalence of diabetes. Estimates for the year 2000 and projections for 2030. Diabetes Care 2004;27:1047-53.

World Health Organization. Definition and diagnosis of diabetes mellitus and intermediate hypoglycaemia: report of a WHO/IDF consultation. WHO Geneva. 2006. http://www.who.int/diabetes/publications/Definition%20and%20diagnosis%20of%20diabetes_new.pdf

Diabetes Mellitus
Top Ten
International Diabetes Federation. Diabetes Atlas http://www.eatlas.idf.org/

Obesity
International Obesity Task Force http://www.iotf.org/

Diabetes Trends
International Diabetes Federation.

50–51 MENTAL HEALTH
World Health Organization. The world health report 2006: Working together for health. Geneva: WHO; 2006.

World Health Organization. Human resources and training in mental health. Geneva: WHO; 2005.

World Health Organization. Promoting mental health: concepts, emerging evidence, practice. Geneva: WHO; 2005.

World Health Organization. Mental health atlas: 2005. Geneva: WHO; 2005.

World Health Organization. Prevention of mental disorders: effective interventions and policy options. Geneva: WHO; 2004.

Suicide Rates
World Health Organization Department of Mental Health and Substance Abuse http://www.who.int/mental_health/prevention/suicide_rates/en/index.htm

Major Mental Disorders
World Health Organization. Disease control priorities related to mental, neurological, developmental and substance abuse disorders. Geneva: WHO; 2006. Available at: http://www.dcp2.org

Care in the Community
World Health Organization. Mental health atlas: 2005. op. cit. p17

52–53 VIOLENCE AND ABUSE
World Health Organization. World report on violence and health. Geneva: WHO; 2002.

Garcia-Morena C, Jansen HAFM, Ellsberg M, Heise L, Watts C. Prevalence of intimate partner violence: findings from the World Health Organization multi-country study on women's health and domestic violence. Lancet 2006;368:1260-9.

Murder
World Health Organization. 2002. op. cit.

Murder of Children
World Health Organization. Global estimates of health consequences due to violence against children. Background paper to the UN Secretary General's Study on Violence against Children. 2006.

Violence against Women by Intimate Partner
Garcia-Morena C et al. 2006. op. cit.
Japan is unweighted data. Rest of data is "weighted for number of eligible women in household".

Female Genital Mutilation/Cutting
UNICEF. The state of the world's children 2007. New York: UNICEF; 2006. Table 9.

54–55 INJURY

World Health Organization. Preventing injuries and violence: a guide for ministries of health. Geneva: WHO; 2007.

World Health Organization. World report on road traffic injury prevention. Geneva: WHO; 2004.

World Health Organization. World report on violence and health. Geneva: WHO; 2002.

Fatal Road Crashes
World Bank resources. http://siteresources.worldbank. org/EXTROADSAFETY/Resources/graph13.x

Deaths per 100,000 people
WHO Global Burden of Disease Estimates. Table 5. Age standardized death rates per 100,000 by cause and member state (2002) Available at: http://www.who.int/

WHO 2004. op. cit. Table A4.

WHO 2002 op. cit. Table A8.

Deaths from Injury
WHO 2002. op. cit.

The Injury Chart Book http://whqlibdoc.who.int/ publications/924156220X.pdf

56–57 RESPIRATORY DISEASES

Chapman KR, Mannino DM, Soriano JB et al. Epidemiology and costs of chronic obstructive pulmonary disease. Eur Resp J 2006;27:188-207.

Lopez AD, Shibuya K, Rao C et al. Chronic obstructive pulmonary disease: current burden and future projections. Eur Resp J 2006;27:397-412.

Rehfuess E, Mehta S, Pruss-Ustun A. Assessing household solid fuel use: Multiple implications for the Millennium Development Goals. Environ Health Perspect 2006;114:272-378.

Pneumonia
Under-fives taken to health facilities
World Health Organization Statistical Information System. http://www.who.int/whosis/

Asthma
Masoli M, Fabian D, Holt S, Beasley R, for the Global Initiative for Asthma (GINA) Programme. The Global Burden of Asthma: executive summary of the GINA Dissemination Committee Report. Allergy 2004;59:469-478.

Deaths from Respiratory Conditions
World Health Organization. The top 10 causes of death. http://www.who.int/mediacentre/factsheets/fs310/en/ index.html (accessed 7 October 2007)

58–59 DIARRHOEAL DISEASES

UNDP. Human Development Report 2006. New York: UNDP; 2006. Available at: http://hdr.undp.org/hdr2006/

World Health Organization. World Health Statistics 2007. Geneva: WHO; 2007.

Thapar N, Sanderson IR. Diarrhoea in Children: an interface between developed and developing countries. Lancet 2004;363:641-653.

Fontaine O, Newton C. A revolution in the management of diarrhoea. Bulletin WHO 2001;79:471-2.

Deaths from Diarrhoea
ORT
World Health Organization. op. cit. 2007.

Cholera Pandemic
World Health Organization. Weekly Epidemiological Record http://www.who.int/topics/cholera/surveillance/ en/index.html (accessed 16 September 2007).

60–61 VACCINE-PREVENTABLE DISEASES

World Health Organization. World health statistics 2007. Geneva: WHO; 2007. Table 3.

World Health Organization and UNICEF. Immunization summary: The 2007 Edition. New York: UNICEF; 2007.

World Health Organization/Unicef/World Bank. State of the world's vaccines and immunization. Geneva: WHO; 2002.

Anand S, Berninghausen T. Health workers and vaccination coverage: an econometric analysis. Lancet 2007;369:1277-85.

Measles Vaccination
World Health Organization. 2007 op. cit. Table 3.

Polio
World Health Organization. 2007 op. cit. Table 7.

Changes in Coverage
World Health Organization and UNICEF; 2007. op. cit.

62–63 SEXUALLY TRANSMITTED INFECTIONS

World Health Organization. Global strategy for the prevention and control of sexually transmitted infections 2006-2015. Geneva: WHO; 2007. Available at: http://www.who.int/

World Health Organization. Global prevalence and incidence of selected curable sexually transmitted infections: overview and estimates. Geneva: WHO; 2001. Available at: http://www.who.int/

UNAIDS/WHO Global HIV/AIDS Online Database. Available at: http://www.who.int/

Curable STIs
World Health Organization. 2001. op. cit.

Condom Use
World Health Organization Statistical Information System. http://www.who.int/whosis/

64–65 HIV/AIDS

UNAIDS/WHO. 2006 Report on the global AIDS epidemic. http://www.unaids.org/en

Prevalence of HIV Infection
Anti-Retroviral Therapy
UNAIDS/WHO. 2006. op. cit.

66–67 TUBERCULOSIS

World Health Organization. World health statistics 2007. Geneva: WHO; 2007. Available at: http://www.who. int/whosis/

World Health Organization. Global tuberculosis control: Surveillance, planning, financing. World Health Organization report 2007. Geneva: WHO; 2007. Available at: http://www.who.int/

Stop TB Partnership. http://www.stoptb.org

Global Alliance for TB Drug Development. http://www. tballiance.org/home/home.php

TB Prevalence
World Health Organization. World health statistics 2007. op. cit. Table 2.

TB deaths among HIV-positive people
World Health Organization. World health statistics 2007. op. cit. Table 1.

Changes in TB
World Health Organization. Global tuberculosis control. 2007 op. cit. Fig 22, p38 and Table A2.1

68–69 MALARIA
World Health Organization. World malaria report 2005. http://rbm.who.int/wmr2005/index.html

World Bank. Rolling Back Malaria. Global strategy and booster programme. Washington DC: World Bank; 2005. Available at: http://www.worldbank.org/

Roll Back Malaria Partnership, Roll Back Malaria Global Malaria Database http://www.rollbackmalaria.org/links.html

Child Deaths from Malaria
World Health Organization. World Health Statistics 2007. Geneva: WHO; 2007. Table 1.

Anti-malarial treatment
Insecticide-treated nets
World Health Organization. World Health Statistics 2007. Geneva: WHO; 2007. Table 3. Available at: http://www.who.int/whosis/

Malaria Transmission and Prevention
Adapted from: World Health Organization. Malaria vector control and personal protection: Report of a WHO study group. WHO technical report series no 936. Geneva: WHO; 2006.
Available at: http://www.who.int/

70–71 Part 4 Public Health Challenges

Population Change
Department of Economic and Social Affairs: Population Division. World population prospects: the 2006 revision. Tables A2, A10.

72–73 URBANIZATION
United Nations Human Settlements programme (UN-Habitat). The challenge of slums: global report on human settlements 2003. London: Earthscan; 2003. http://www.unhabitat.org/pmss/getPage.asp?page=booKView&book=1156

UNICEF. The state of the world's children 2006: Excluded and invisible. New York: UNICEF; 2006.

United Nations Population Fund. State of World Population 2007. Unleashing the potential of urban growth. New York: UNFPA; 2007. http://www.unfpa.org/swp/2007/english/chapter_2/slums.html

Urban Dwellers
World Health Organization Statistical Information System http://www.who.int/whosis/

Megacities
United Nations Department of Economic and Social Affairs, Population Division. World urbanization prospects: The 2005 revision. Available at: http://www.un.org/esa/

Urbanization
World Urbanization Prospects: The 2005 Revisions. Fact Sheet 3. Available at: http://www.un.org/esa/

Changing Urban Population
UN-Habitat. 2003. op. cit.

74–75 CLIMATE CHANGE
Intergovernmental Panel on Climate Change. Working Group II. Climate change impacts, Adaptation and vulnerability. Chapter 8. Human Health. http://www.ipcc-wg2.org/index.html

McMichael AJ, Campbell-Lendrum DH, Corvalan CF et al. editors. Climate change and human health. risk and responses. Geneva: WHO; 2003. Available at: http://www.who.int/

Extreme Weather Events
McMichael AJ. 2003 op. cit. p92.

Adverse Effects on Health of Changes in Temperature and Rainfall
McMichael AJ. 2003 op. cit. p136.

76–77 WAR
Levy BS, Sidel VW. War and Public Health. New York: Oxford University Press; 1997.

Global Health Watch 2005-2006. An alternative world health report. London: Zed Books; London 2005 (in association with People's Health Movement, Bangalore, Medact, London, Global Equity Gauge Alliance, Durban.)

World Health Organization. The World Health Report 2007: A safer future: global public health security in the 21st century. Geneva: WHO; 2007. Available at: Available at: http://www.who.int/

People of Concern to the UNHCR
United Nations High Commission for Refugees. http://www.unhcr.org/statistics.html

Political Violence
World Bank and Human Security Report Project: Miniatlas of human security. Washington DC and Vancouver, BC: World Bank and Human Security Report Project; 2008:32-33. Available at: http://www.miniatlasofhumansecurity.info

Military vs Health Spending
UNDP. Human Development Report 2006. New York: UNDP; 2006. Table 19. Available at: http://hdr.undp.org/hdr2006/

Battle-Deaths
Centre for the Study of Civil War. International Peace Research Institute Norway. http://new.prio.no

Gleditsch NP, Wallensteen P, Eriksson M et al. Armed conflict 1946-2001: A new dataset. Journal of Peace Research 2002;39(5):615-637.

78–79 PANDEMICS
World Health Organization. WHO global influenza preparedness plan. Geneva: WHO; 2005. Available at: http://www.who.int

Avian Influenza H5N1
Death Rate
Cumulative number of confirmed human cases of avian influenza A/(H5N1) Reported to WHO (to 10 September 2007) http://www.who.int/csr/disease/avian_influenza/country/en/

Severe Acute Respiratory Syndrome (SARS)
Death Rate
World Health Organization. Summary table of areas that experienced local transmission of SARS during the outbreak period from 1 November 2002 to 31 July 2003. http://www.who.int/csr/sars/areas/areas2003_11_21/en/index.html

Summary of probable SARS cases 1 November 2002 to 31 July 2003 (posted 21 April 2004) http://www.who.int/csr/sars/country/table2004_04_21/en/index.html

Phases of Pandemic Alert
Current phase of alert in the WHO Global Influenza Preparedness Plan http://www.who.int/csr/disease/avian_influenza/phase/en/index.html

80–81 ANTIMICROBIAL RESISTANCE
World Health Organization. WHO global strategy for the containment of antimicrobial Resistance. Geneva: WHO; 2001.

MDR-TB
World Health Organization. Global tuberculosis control. Surveillance, planning, financing. WHO Report 2007 Geneva: WHO; 2007. Available at: http://www.who.int/

MRSA
Grundmann H, Aires-de-Sousa M, Boyce J, Tiemersma E. Emergence and resurgence of methicillin-resistant *Staphylococcus aureus* as a public health threat. Lancet 2006;368:874-85.

Chloroquine-Resistant Malaria
World Bank Disease Control Priorities Project http://www.dcp2.org/pubs/DCP/55/Figure/55.3

82–83 DISABILITY
DISTAT
http://unstats.un.org/unsd/demographic/sconcerns/disability/disab2.asp

Robert Metts. Disability and Development. Background paper prepared for the Disability and Development Research Agenda Meeting, November 16 2004, World Bank Headquarters, Washington DC. Available at: http://siteresources.worldbank.org

Mont D. Measuring disability prevalence. SP Discussion paper no. 0706. Washington DC: World Bank; 2007. Available at: http://siteresources.worldbank.org

World Health Assembly 2005, Resolutions and descisions. http://www.who.int/gb/ebwha/pdf_files/WHA58/WHA58_23-en.pdf

Collecting the Data
United Nations Statistics Division. Human functioning and disability. http://unstats.un.org/

Blindness
World Health Organization 2002. Global update of available data on visual impairment. Available at: http://www.who.int

Major Causes of Disability
GDP Lost
Robert Metts, 2004 op. cit. p15.

The Framework for the International Classification of Functioning, Disability and Health
Robert Metts, 2004 op. cit. p4.

84–85 AGEING
Butler, RN. Population ageing and health. BMJ 1997;315:1082-4.

Holliday R. Ageing in the 21st century. Lancet 1999;354;SIV4.

Help Age International. The ageing and development report: Poverty, independence and the world's older people. London: Earthscan; 1999.

World Health Organization. Active ageing: A policy framework. Geneva: WHO; 2002.

Elderly Population
United Nations Department of Economic and Social Affairs, Population Division. World population prospects. The 2006 revision. Highlights, Working paper no. ESA/P/WP.202. Table A10. Available at: http://www.un.org/esa

Ageing Populations
United Nations Department of Economic and Social Affairs, 2006. op. cit. Table 1.3.

Potential Support Ratio
United Nations Department of Economic and Social Affairs. World Population Ageing 2007. Figure II. Available at: http://www.un.org/esa/

85–86 UNHEALTHY DIETS
World Health Organization. Global strategy on diet, physical activity and health. Geneva: WHO; 2004. Available at: http://www.who.int/

Joint WHO/FAO Expert consultation on diet, nutrition and the prevention of chronic diseases: Report of a joint WHO/FAO expert consultation, Geneva, 28 January-1 February 2002. WHO technical report series; 916. WHO, Geneva 2003. http://whqlibdoc.who.int/trs/WHO_TRS_916.pdf

World Health Organization. Globalization, diets and noncommunicable diseases. Geneva: WHO; 2002. http://whqlibdoc.who.int/publications/9241590416.pdf

International Obesity Task Force http://www.iotf.org/globalepidemic.asp

United Nations Standing Committee on Nutrition. The fifth report on the world nutrition situation: Nutrition for improved development outcomes. SCN; 2004.

UNICEF. The state of the world's children 2007. New York: UNICEF; 2006.

World Health Organization. WHO Global strategy for food safety. WHO, Geneva 2002. Available at: http://www.who.int/

Underweight Children
UNDP. Human Development Report 2006. New York: UNDP; 2006. Available at: http://hdr.undp.org/hdr2006/

No Progress
Food and Agriculture Organization of the United Nations. The state of food insecurity in the world 2006. Rome: FAO. 2006. Table 1 Available at: http://www.fao.org/

Overweight Children
SCN 2004. op. cit.

Changing Diet in Rural China
National Bureau of Statistics of China. Available at: http://www.stats.gov.cn/english/statisticaldata/yearlydata/

88–89 HUMAN RESOURCES
World Health Organization. World health report 2006: Working together for health. Geneva: WHO; 2006.

Joint Learning Initiative. Human resources for health. Overcoming the crisis. Global Equity Initiative, Harvard University. 2004.

Healthcare Staff
World Health Organization. World health statistics 2007. Geneva: WHO; 2007.

Impact of Health Workers
Brain Drain
World Health Organization. World health report 2006: Working together for health. Geneva: WHO; 2006.

90–91 HEALTH RESEARCH

Global Forum for Health Research. http://www.globalforumhealth.org/Site/000__Home.php

Commission on Health Research for Development http://www.cohred.org/main/

COHRED's Human Resources for Health Research Initiative http://www.cohred.org/HR-HR/Human_Resources_Health_more.htm

Nuyens Y. No development without research. Global Forum for Health Research, Geneva 2005. Available at: http://www.globalforumhealth.org/

De Francisco A & Matlin S (eds). Monitoring financial flows for health research 2006: The changing landscape of health research for development. Global Forum for Health Research. Geneva 2006. Available at: http://www.globalforumhealth.org/

De Francisco A. The Global Forum for Health Research. Presentation at meeting of the Western Pacific ACHR & Health Research Councils, 4 October 2005, slide 25. Available at: http://www.wpro.who.int/

Published Research

Rahman M, Fukui T. Biomedical publication – global profile and trend. Public Health 2003;117:274-80.

De Francisco A & Matlin S. 2006. op. cit.

Growth of Expenditure
Distribution of Expenditure

De Francisco A & Matlin S. 2006. op cit.

92–93 MEASURING HEALTH

World Health Organization. Surveillance of noncommunicable disease risk factors. Factsheet No 273. http://www.who.int/mediacentre/factsheets/fs273/en/

Health Metrics Network http://www.who.int/healthmetrics/en/

Mathers CD, Ma Fat D, Inoue M, Rao C, Lopez AD. Counting the dead and what they died from: An assessment of the global status of death data. Bulletin WHO 2005;83:171-7.

Hill, K. Making deaths count. Bulletin World Health Organization 2006;84:162.

Shibuya K. Counting the dead is essential for health. Bulletin World Health Organization 2006;84:170-1.

Death Registration
Pattern of Disease

World Health Organization Statistical Information System http://www.who.int/whosis/

Age of Death

World Health Organization. The Top Ten Causes of Death. Fact Sheet No 310 http://www.who.int/mediacentre/factsheets/fs310/en/index1.html

94–95 Part 5 Dates, Definitions and Data

Maternal Mortality Ratio

WHO. World Health Organization Statistics 2007. Geneva: WHO; 2007. p10. Available at: http://www.who.int/

96–99 SIGNIFICANT EVENTS IN PUBLIC HEALTH

Centers for Disease Control http://www.cdc.gov/

Mackay J, Jemal A, Lee NC, Parkin DM. The cancer atlas. Atlanta: American Cancer Society; 2006.

McKeown T. The origins of human disease. Oxford: Basil Blackwell; 1988.

Porter R. The greatest benefit to mankind. A medical history of humanity from antiquity to the present. London: Harper Collins;1997

102–09 HEALTH PROBLEMS

1 Health Problems

Life expectancy; Maternal deaths: UNICEF. The state of the world's children 2007. New York: UNICEF; 2006.

Under-five deaths; Cancer deaths; CVD deaths; Deaths of under-fives (pneumonia; diarrhoea; malaria); Measles; Tuberculosis: WHOSIS

Diabetes: International Diabetes Federation. Diabetes Atlas http://www.eatlas.idf.org/

HIV/AIDS: 2006 Report on the global AIDS epidemic. UNAIDS/WHO 2006.

110–17 DETERMINANTS & CHALLENGES

Population; Gross National Income; Education: UNICEF. The state of the world's children 2007. New York: UNICEF; 2006.

Population aged 60 or over: UN Department of Economic and Social Affairs, World Population Ageing 2007. New York: UNDP; 2007. Table A.III.4.

Inequality ratio; Healthcare spending; Water, Sanitation; Underweight under-fives: UNDP Human Development Report 2006. New York: UNDP; 2006.

Healthcare staff; Overweight under-fives; Alcohol: WHOSIS.

Nutrition: FAO statistical database.

Tobacco: Mackay, J. et al. The Cancer Atlas. Atlanta, Georgia: American Cancer Society. 2006.

Photo Credits

32 Jimmy Wong; 75 Mark Lynas; 83 iStockphoto/Kenneth C Zirkel; 80 iStockphoto/Douglas Allen; 89 WHO/Carlos Gaggero.

Whilst every reasonable effort has been made to contact the copyright holders for images used in the atlas, the authors and publisher will gladly receive information that will enable them to rectify any inadvertent errors in subsequent editions.

INDEX

gender difference in:
- access to education 9, 26–27, 30
- access to ARV therapy 64
- access to services 18
- elderly populations 84
- employment 30, 34–35
- HIV rates 10
- urban environment 72

gonorrhoea 62–63
Gross Domestic Product (GDP)
- lost to disability 82
- lost to malaria 68

Gross National Income (GNI) 24–25

Haemophilius influenzae type B (Hib) vaccine 60
health
- data 10, 24, 44, 82–83, 92–93, 95
- definition of 9
- research 66, 80, 90–91, 95
- surveillance systems 10, 11, 66, 68, 74, 80, 92, 95

health workers 71, 88–89
healthcare 16, 36–37, 76, 84
- access to 18, 32, 36
- for ALRI 56–57
- government spending on 36, 76, 77, 88
- impact of malaria on 68
- inequality of access to 37, 72
- preventive measures 36
- primary 12, 36, 50, 66, 84
- privatization of 11
- rehabilitation and support 82
- sexual and reproductive 62
- unaffordable 18

heart disease 28, 32, 46–47 *see also* cardiovascular disease
hepatitis 40, 44, 60, 62
heroin 40–41
herpes 62
high blood pressure 46, *see also* hypertension
HIV/AIDS 16, 26, 40, 58, 62, 64–65, 91, 99
- and effect on health workers 88
- and mental health 50
- and tuberculosis 66–67
- anti-retroviral (ARV) therapy 64, 65, 88, 99
- impact on education 26, 64
- impact on life expectancy 17
- in slum areas 72
- under-fives 20, 21
- vaccine, search for 60, 64

housing 16, 32–33, 84

hospital beds 36
human papilloma virus (HPV) 44, 62
- vaccine 60

Human Poverty Index 24–25
human rights 11, 82
hygiene 30
hypertension 46

illiteracy 9, 26
immunization 20, 43 *see also* vaccine-preventable diseases 60–61

inequality 10, 23, 24–25, 97
- and effect on health 24
- and mental illness 50
- Black report on 99
- child health 20, 25, 26
- gender 10, 26–27, 18, 30, 34–35, 64, 72
- in access to health services 20, 37, 50, 60
- in access to malaria programmes 68
- in access to safe water 30
- in educational attainment 26
- of health outcomes 28, 43

Inequality Ratio 24
inequity 10, 13
infant
- HIV infection 64
- measles vaccination 60–61
- mortality rate 9 24–25, 26
- perinatal conditions 43

infection-control practices 80
infectious diseases *see* communicable diseases
influenza
- pandemic 78
- vaccination 60

injury 42, 54–55
- and alcohol use 40
- cause of death in young people 54, 55
- death from 43, 54–55
- domestic 32
- intentional 52, 54, 76
- occupational 34, 35
- unintentional 54–55

insecticide-treated bednets (ITN) 20, 68–69
International Bill of Human Rights 9, 11
International Classification of Functioning, Disability and Health 82, 83
International Health Regulations 79, 99

life expectancy 9, 15, 16–17, 46, 71, 84
literacy, impact on education 26
living conditions 9, 15, 32–33, 72–73, 82

malaria 68–69, 91, 96, 97
- climate-related 74–75
- diarrhoeal diseases 58
- drug resistance 68, 80–81
- impact on education 26
- under-fives 20, 21
- vaccine, search for 60, 68

malnutrition 9, 28–29, 71
- and diarrhoea 28, 58
- and disability 82
- climate-related 74–75
- in migrating populations 76
- in under-fives 20, 21, 26, 28, 56
- in urban environments 72
- transmission and prevention 69

maternal health 18–19, 28
- and FGM 52

maternal mortality 15, 18–19, 26, 43, 71, 94
- and education 18
- and literacy 18
- causes of 19

measles
- diarrhoeal diseases 58
- in migrating populations 76
- in under-fives 20, 21
- vaccination 60–61

mental health problems 34, 50–51
- alcohol and 40

methicillin-resistant *Staphylococcus aureus* (MRSA) 80–81
micronutrient supplements 20
migrating populations 11
- caused by climate change 75
- caused by war or violence 52, 76–77
- rural to urban 32, 72–73
- vulnerability to malaria 68

military, government spending on 11, 37, 77
Millennium Development Goals 60, 99
murder 52, 53

neonatal deaths 20, 21
non-communicable diseases 15, 28, 34, 38, 40, 43, 44, 46, 48, 50, 71, 84, 86, 90
non-governmental organizations 36